The Slimming Foodie

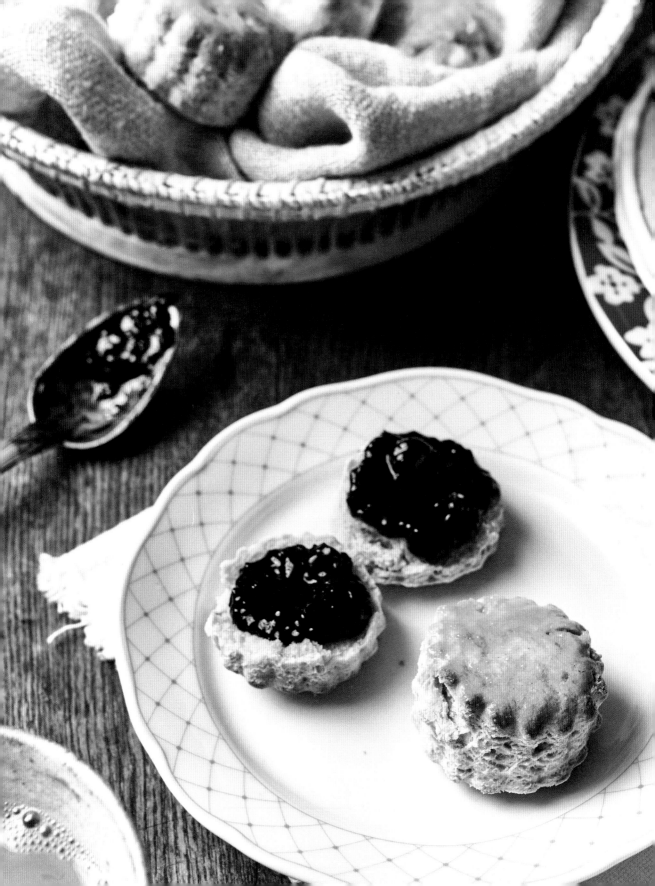

The Slimming Foodie

PIP PAYNE

aster

First published in Great Britain in 2021 by Aster,
an imprint of Octopus Publishing Group Ltd
Carmelite House
50 Victoria Embankment
London EC4Y 0DZ
www.octopusbooks.co.uk

An Hachette UK Company
www.hachette.co.uk

ISBN 978 1 78325 416 3

A CIP catalogue record for this book is available from
the British Library.

Printed and bound in Italy by Printer Trento S.r.l.

10 9 8 7 6 5 4

Commissioning Editor: Natalie Bradley
Senior Managing Editor: Sybella Stephens
Copy Editor: Lucy Bannell
Art Director: Yasia Williams-Leedham
Designers: Peter Dawson and Amy Shortis at gradedesign.com
Photographer: Chris Terry
Food Stylist: Henrietta Clancy
Props Stylist: Tamsin Weston
Assistant Production Manager: Lucy Carter

Author's notes:

The information contained in this book is not intended to replace any dietary advice from your own qualified nutrition-ist or dietician. Any application of the ideas and information contained in this book is at the reader's sole discretion and risk.

Both imperial and metric measurements have been given in all recipes. Use one set of measurements only and not a mixture of both.

 Vegetarian

 Slow-cooker recipe

 The most popular recipes from The Slimming Foodie blog

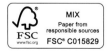

CONTENTS

INTRODUCTION

I grew up in Torbay in South Devon, UK, with two very different food influences. The first, naturally, was my parents, who had met and worked in France in the 1970s and possessed unusually continental tastes for my 1980s childhood. They were excited to share their love of French cheeses, Italian meats and Greek salads with my brother and me – all the amazing foods that they hadn't experienced in their post-war childhoods. To their disappointment, I was an incredibly fussy eater. My mum's first breakthrough with me was that she discovered I would eat almost any vegetable if it was in a curry! The second was my grandma. Her way of cooking was morning fry-ups, steak pie and baked beans, roast dinners, cottage pies… good, hearty, stodgy comfort food which always made me happy.

I've always loved to cook. My mum set an example by cooking from scratch, encouraging me to learn to cook and be responsible for feeding the family at least once a week.

When I left school, I developed a fresh appreciation of food and cuisines from other countries, travelling through France and Italy, Mexico and Central America, trying new flavours and combinations of ingredients. One of my favourite things about travelling is visiting food markets, or even supermarkets, seeing the astonishing variety, eating and discovering local food. In Thailand I experienced sitting by the beach on a humid, balmy evening, with a steaming, fragrant bowl of tom yum soup – it's amazing how spicy food can be so refreshing. I loved the huge knobbly lemons and wedges of Parmesan in the supermarkets in Italy. It's incredible that even motorway service stations there serve amazing pizza, reminiscent of the slices you can buy in the back streets of Rome. Volunteering for the morning breakfast run on family holidays to France is a real treat for me, visiting the boulangerie for crusty baguettes and warm *pains au chocolat*. Experiencing street food in Mexico is one of my favourite food memories – spicy tacos, quesadillas and steaming refried beans – and I've so enjoyed trying to recreate these flavours at home.

I love food. I love shopping for it, cooking it, eating it and sharing it. Looking, smelling, tasting and experimenting with food brings me a huge amount of joy. I love to experiment when cooking, tasting as I go along, and I encourage every cook to do the same, to see how flavours change…just the addition of a single spice can make a meal pop.

I discovered a love of bringing friends together around the table during my first flatshare in London with friends. I enjoyed playing 'mother hen' and keeping everyone fed. After a night out, we would come home to a slow cooker bubbling with beef and ale casserole instead of a takeaway.

As life and work got busier, I met my husband and we had our first daughter. I adapted my way of cooking to save on time, and started to embrace batch cooking and other ways to keep eating well when there was little time to cook. We moved from London back to Devon in 2012, when I was pregnant with my second daughter.

In Devon we have a lot of incredible independent food producers, from fruit and vegetable suppliers to our local dairy. I enjoy visiting farm shops and markets to experience all the amazing produce, but that isn't always practical for day-to-day life, so I often shop at supermarkets to get everything I need in one place. With this in mind, I've made sure the ingredients in this book are easily available at the supermarket, but I encourage you to explore local food options too. It's exciting to discover new ingredients and incorporate them into your cooking.

I started The Slimming Foodie blog in 2015. My two daughters were aged five and two, and after both of my pregnancies, a big move from London to Devon, and starting a new business with my husband, I had gained a lot of weight. I didn't feel fit or healthy, I had lost my self-confidence, and sleepless nights and stress led me to seek comfort in food. I had reached a point where my weight was seriously affecting my happiness, and I knew I had to take steps to change things before it affected my health too.

Searching the internet for healthy, slimming recipes, I just wasn't inspired. I didn't want to eat 'diet food' and I didn't want to lose my enjoyment of eating. I still wanted to look forward to every meal and I knew that I needed to find a way of cooking that would allow me to do that. I started taking my favourite recipes and adjusting them to make them healthier: using more vegetables, cutting down on added fats and sugars, finding healthy swaps, and avoiding processed and pre-packaged food. I started a Facebook page, sharing a quick snap of my dinner and attaching the recipe. It felt like a good way to keep a casual diary of what I was eating, share recipe successes and failures and hold myself accountable. It quickly grew in popularity, so I set up the blog to make the recipes available to anyone looking for healthy cooking inspiration. The meals were – and still are – easy for a novice home cook to achieve, dishes that anyone would be happy to eat regularly: good, balanced, delicious food that just happens to be slimming. The most popular recipes from my blog are highlighted with a star in the book.

Food shouldn't be tied up with guilt and shame, it should be a positive and enjoyable thing. I also don't think that the word 'slimming' should hold a negative connotation. Slimming is a personal choice, and it's an empowering decision to make. Knowing that you need to make a change, as I did, should be celebrated and supported, and I hope this book helps anyone on that journey. Losing weight is not easy and there isn't a quick fix that is sustainable. It requires a long-term lifestyle change, involving both healthy eating and increased physical activity. Weight is very much entwined with mental health too. It's a complex issue, and I hope that by offering these tasty, fun, enjoyable and varied recipes, I can make the home cooking part of the process a little bit easier.

MY THOUGHTS ON HEALTHY EATING

There are so many misleading messages around healthy eating and dieting, with new fads emerging all the time. I've always kept up to date with science-based food news and I adopt a common sense approach to healthy eating. I eat a varied, balanced diet, based around the principle of moderation in all things. Cutting down on added fats and sugars where I can, I try to put more vegetables, fruits, pulses and legumes on my plate, as well as good proteins, such as fish, eggs, poultry, red meat, nuts and seeds. I increase my fibre intake wherever possible too. By avoiding processed and pre-packaged convenience foods, I know exactly what I am eating, while keeping indulgent foods and drinks as an occasional treat means I don't feel that I'm missing out.

It's simple enough, but healthy food starts with cooking from scratch. Processed foods, ready-made meals and takeaways are often stuffed with unnecessary extra calories and salt. If you want to have a healthy diet, you need to embrace the joy of cooking! I know this isn't always easy – work, family and household pressures can make it seem that you don't have time to spend in the kitchen – but there are a few things you can do to help make home cooking a little easier:

1. **Plan a weekly menu and shop accordingly.** Knowing what you are going to be cooking takes away the exhausting evening storecupboard raids to try to find something to cook.

2. **Make the most of healthy convenience foods that have been prepared for you.** Embrace pre-chopped onions, frozen chopped butternut squash, frozen cod fillets…there's no shame in using these to make life easier and quicker.

3. **Batch cook.** If I'm cooking something that will freeze well (such as Rustic Devonshire Pork in Cider, Weekend Veggie Chilli or Slow-cooker Mexican Beef (see pages 121, 157 and 180), I'll often try to cook extra so I have some to freeze – homemade ready meals when you need them! (For the best freezer-friendly meals in this book, see page 218.)

4. **Use a slow cooker.** If you can find 10 minutes in the morning, you can throw together a slow-cooker meal such as Slow-cooker Honey Garlic Chicken or Chinese Pulled Pork (see pages 66 and 179) that will be ready and waiting when you get home.

5. **Try to relax about cooking.** Instead of seeing it as a chore, put some music on and enjoy the process. It's a great activity to take your mind off other worries and has the added benefit of nourishing your body.

ABOUT THIS BOOK

I am a home cook, not a chef, which helps me to understand what's achievable and realistic at home. The recipes in this book are true to how I cook. I look for ways to simplify dishes and save time, always keeping in mind a great-tasting final dish that can be happily shared with family and friends, without anyone having an inkling that it's healthy or slimming.

It's important to start the day with a good breakfast, so in the first chapter you'll find some ideas that you can make up the night before or quickly put together at the start of the day. But don't worry, I haven't forgotten about those lazy weekend breakfasts either.

Quick & Easy Midweek Meals are for those days when you're running around like crazy and just need a dish that won't take long to put together, but still delivers on flavour.

When I have friends coming over, I like something I can get ready in advance and not spend a lot of time tending to – this is where One-pot Wonders and Savoury Traybakes come in. There's something so satisfying about putting all the ingredients in one pot and letting them come together.

The Family Favourites chapter has winning ideas for meals that everyone can enjoy, and these can be easily adapted for fussy eaters.

We all know it's important to increase our vegetable intake and I look for easy ways to do this in the Light Dishes & Sides chapter. I've also included some of my favourite super-quick veggie side dishes that you can prepare in advance and have ready in the refrigerator, or that take a short time to make.

Eating in a balanced way, it's still really important to treat yourself, and I love having something that feels a bit more indulgent at the weekend – my Friday Night Specials will rival any takeaway.

In the Simple Bakes & Desserts chapter, I've included some of my go-to baked goods, including a family recipe for a quick no-knead bread and a few easy ideas for some tasty (but lower calorie) cakes.

A good array of herbs and spices is really key to tasty, lower calorie cooking, so I have included spice mixes in the last chapter. For each of the spice mixes you will find corresponding meals that are extra quick and easy once you have your spice blend ready (of course, if you haven't had a chance to make up the spice mixes, you can buy spice blends from the supermarket).

I've also included ideas for how to use up leftover vegetables, make homemade stocks and get the most out of ingredients, as well as ideas for batch cooking for the freezer. You'll also find suggestions throughout the book on how to use up other leftovers.

Anyone should be able to cook these recipes, no matter what your kitchen ability, so I've made sure that all the ingredients are easy to source and the techniques used in the methods are straightforward.

MY STORECUPBOARD, REFRIGERATOR & FREEZER

There are some ingredients that I always like to have in the house, so I can whip up a tasty, healthy meal without having to go to the shops. When I do a weekly shop, I try and choose some vegetables with a reasonably long shelf life, so I can cook with them all week. These are the key ingredients I usually have in:

STORECUPBOARD
Vegetables, fruit & herbs
Sweet potatoes & butternut squash: Both have a long shelf life, are quite robust when cooked and add a natural sweetness to dishes. They are so versatile to use in curries, traybakes, quiches and hummus, and are great for vegetarian cooking too.

Onions: I always keep red and brown onions stocked up, as they form the basis of so many great meals. When kept in a cool, dark place, they last 2–3 months.

Shallots: With a milder taste than onions, these are lovely for adding a more subtle flavour to dishes, and are great added into casseroles or simply roasted.

Spring onions: Easy and quick to prepare, these add attractive greenness to dishes and, when raw, a much less overwhelming flavour than regular onion.

Garlic: Brings amazing flavour to so many dishes. I always try and select bulbs that have nice big cloves, as I find them much less fiddly to peel.

Ginger: A key ingredient for lots of curries and soups.

Carrots: These have a long shelf life and are useful in many dishes, and make a great soup if you're low on ingredients. You can also pickle them to make them last even longer.

Broccoli: Quick to cook, this goes with most dishes. Don't throw away the stalks! They are sweet and delicious in stir-fries and soup (see page 143).

Asparagus: I just love the flavour and tenderness of these spears, which are wonderful unadorned. They are simple and quick to cook, and great for quiches too.

Cherry tomatoes: Ideal for salads, quick pasta dishes and roasting. Where possible, try and buy them on the vine, as they are so much more flavoursome. You can also roast them on the vine, which looks great on the plate.

Peppers: With a long shelf life, these can be used both raw and cooked, and work well in lots of recipes. Red, yellow and orange peppers are the sweetest, while green have a more bitter flavour that works really well in certain dishes.

Celery: Adds great depth as a base for lots of dishes.

Leeks: These add great oneony background flavour and are very versatile. Always make sure to give them a thorough wash.

Spinach: A good-value ingredient ideal for adding to curries, soups, stews and salads.

Mushrooms: Quick to cook and with a meaty texture, these are always handy to have around. Supermarkets now tend to stock a wide variety, so it's worth experimenting.

Lemons, limes & oranges: The zest and juice of citrus fruit is ideal for adding fresh and bright flavours to food.

Raspberries, blueberries & strawberries: I like to have fresh berries for breakfasts and snacks. Although they have a short shelf life, raspberries and blueberries can be frozen if you haven't eaten them all within a couple of days.

Chillies: Lots of varieties offering different heat levels and flavours that can really make a difference to a dish. Scotch bonnets, for example, although very hot, also have a delicious, unique sweet taste and really stand out in the puttanesca sauce that I cook at home (see page 62).

Herbs: Key to enhancing flavour in meals, a fresh herb garnish can make an amazing difference both to taste and presentation. I mainly use parsley, basil, mint and coriander, but I also love the flavours of rosemary, sage and thyme. To save waste, it really makes sense to keep potted herbs, or plant them in the garden. Mint, rosemary, sage and thyme are incredibly hardy outside

and don't need much maintenance. I keep basil and parsley potted on the kitchen windowsill and these last well, as long as you remember to water them…

Grains, seeds & pasta

Oats: These are perfect for filling breakfasts such as baked oats, and even cakes, with the added bonus that they are high in fibre. I buy jumbo oats for porridge, as they are more robust and hold their shape and texture, while I use cheaper, regular porridge oats for baking and overnight oats.

Basmati rice: Great as a quick side dish for a curry or a casserole.

Brown rice: I love the slightly more chewy texture of brown rice, and it's ideal for a filling side dish. Brown rice is also a great swap for white rice, for its increased fibre levels.

Wholewheat couscous: So quick when you are in a hurry, this makes a great side dish for almost anything. I can't really taste the difference between wholewheat and white couscous, so I would rather benefit from the added fibre in the wholewheat version.

Quinoa: A fantastic high-protein, wheat-free option that works well in salads and as a side dish.

Bulgur wheat: Quick to cook and a fantastic base for salads.

Spaghetti: Great for a quick meal. It's really important not to overcook spaghetti – retain a slight bite so it doesn't end up stodgy.

Orzo: Perfect for bulking up soups and

making traybakes, this rice-shaped pasta is now readily available in most supermarkets.

Chia seeds: I love the texture that these can add to a wet ingredient such as yogurt – both thickening it and giving a slight bite – and when baking they add a satisfying crunchiness.

Sunflower seeds: Useful for adding a little crunch and texture to a savoury dish. I tend to use these instead of pine nuts as they are much better value and very readily available.

Cans, bottles & jars

Canned tomatoes: I use these all the time for brilliant pasta sauces, rich stews and curries.

Tomato purée: A great way of thickening and adding richness to curries and casseroles.

Canned pulses: Chickpeas, black beans, pinto beans, lentils, cannellini beans, butter beans, haricot beans – these are the building blocks of many quick and easy snacks and meals, such as soups, stews, hummus and curries. They are great as a nutritious way to make a meal more filling, and of course they have a long shelf life. I also use dried beans and lentils, but you can't beat canned for convenience.

Light coconut milk: A great swap from full-fat coconut milk, as you still get that subtle coconutty flavour and creamy texture.

Soy sauce: A good way to season a dish, this can also add deep colour. I usually keep both light and dark to use in different dishes.

Fish sauce: Although this smells quite pungent, don't let that put you off, as it doesn't carry through into the taste of the final dish, instead providing incredible depth.

Worcestershire sauce: This deepens flavours in savoury sauces and casseroles.

Balsamic and red wine vinegar: Great for roasting vegetables, making dressings and adding depth to sauces.

Anchovies: Perfect for a quick pasta sauce, these add punchy flavour. It's amazing how they disappear into a dish, while adding their savoury saltiness.

Tuna: This can be eaten straight from the can, added to salads, or in a quick pasta dish or bake.

Pesto: You can whip up lots of quick, tasty meals using just a little of this fragrant basil sauce.

Pickled jalapeños: I use these a lot. They add heat and flavour to Mexican dishes and even make a fabulous addition to hummus.

Roasted peppers in brine: Although you can make roasted peppers at home, the process is a little labour intensive so, as these are readily available, I use them regularly for convenience. They have a sweet, rich flavour and a long shelf life.

Spray olive oil: I have a refillable kitchen oil mister, which allows me to control the amount of oil I use and get good coverage on a pan.

Low-calorie cooking spray: I use this for most of my frying and baking, to reduce the added fat in meals.

Wholegrain & Dijon mustards: Useful for flavouring sauces and traybakes and making salad dressings.

Spices, dried herbs & sauces
Spices: Having a good stock of spices can very quickly elevate a meal, creating exciting, flavoursome food. My most commonly used spices are chilli powder, chilli flakes, onion granules, garlic granules, smoked paprika, cumin, turmeric, ground coriander, garam masala, cinnamon and curry powder. Most spices have a good shelf life, but do keep an eye on them as they will lose their flavour over time.

Dried herbs: These can quickly penetrate a dish and bring bold flavour. They are also useful if you don't have any fresh herbs. My most frequently used dried herbs are oregano, thyme, parsley, mixed herbs and Italian seasoning.

Salt & pepper: I like these most of all when they are freshly ground, as it's easy to control the portion and freshly ground pepper often adds the perfect finishing touch to the presentation of a dish too.

Stock pots/cubes: Whether chicken, beef or vegetable, I usually prefer to use stock pots as I think they have more flavour, but sometimes it's useful to have a stock cube to crumble into a sauce. I also use them as a seasoning for roast potatoes.

Sriracha chilli sauce: This is such a versatile ingredient. I use it in sauces, salad dressings, on melted cheese and just to drizzle over food!

Sweet stuff & baking ingredients
Vanilla extract: So useful for adding a natural sweetness and flavour to baking.

Pure maple syrup: I love the unique flavour that this brings, and it's so sweet that you don't need to use much.

Honey: Very useful for a little burst of sweetness, and I adore the caramelized flavours it brings to savoury cooking.

Peanut butter: A rich flavour that enhances both savoury and sweet dishes.

Baking powder: Just a little goes a long way towards making pancakes fluffy.

Wholemeal flour: I always try to use wholemeal flour in baking, for added fibre.

REFRIGERATOR

Fat-free Greek yogurt: One of my most frequently used ingredients. I serve it with berries and granola, add it to baked oats, and use it to replace the oil in hummus or other fats in cakes. It also helps to make a curry creamy and to marinate and tenderize meat.

Eggs: These can be used for so many options for every meal of the day. Try them in a quick frittata for lunch, or fried up with spring onions and chilli to serve with a noodle dish.

Cheddar cheese: Great for a quick lunch such as cheese on toast, but also irresistible served as a melted and bubbling crust on top of a big pot of food.

Parmesan cheese: I love Parmesan grated on top of soups and pastas, and it's a lovely way to add a final flourish when presenting a dish. With its intense flavour, a little goes a long way.

Meats: The meats I use most frequently are chicken thigh fillets, chicken breasts, lean minced beef (less than 5 per cent fat), casserole beef, lamb neck fillets, pork fillet and smoked bacon medallions. I always try to buy the best quality meat that I can, and higher-welfare meat has much better flavour and texture.

FREEZER

Diced onion: Don't knock it until you've tried it! It's perfect for throwing together a slow cooker meal or any kind of curry.

Butternut squash cubes: I find these really handy for saving the prep time on squash, when making a quick curry or stew.

Peas: These go with most meals and are fresh as the day they were picked. You can make a fab quick soup with them too.

Sweetcorn: Perfect as a quick side dish for lots of meals, and a great salad ingredient.

Fruit: Raspberries, blueberries, mango, passion fruit pulp – I use these in overnight oats and baking, or for a quick chia seed jam (see page 25).

Leftovers: My freezer is mainly full of batch-cooked meals, ready to defrost for quick and easy suppers when I need them.

Oven chips: To save waste, I make these myself whenever I have surplus potatoes. Peel some potatoes and cut into chips, then boil for a few minutes, drain and allow to cool. Add salt or spice mixes and coat with low-calorie cooking spray before portioning into freezer bags or airtight containers.

Cod fillets: If I can't get fresh fish from a fishmonger, then I would rather buy it frozen, as it's usually caught and frozen at sea, so you really can't get fresher.

Salmon fillets: A perfect 'hero' ingredient to build a meal around.

ESSENTIAL KITCHEN EQUIPMENT & SUPPLIES

POTS & PANS

Sauté pan: A deep frying pan with a lid is probably my most commonly used pan. It's great for both frying and simmering and big enough to hold a whole meal for 4.

Frying pan: A good, nonstick frying pan is essential when you aren't adding much oil.

Hob-to-oven casserole dish: A big, deep pot with a lid that you can use on the hob and then transfer to the oven is incredibly useful, and provides the perfect way to serve up a meal straight from oven to table.

USEFUL ITEMS

Stainless-steel baking trays: Basic stainless-steel trays are the easiest to clean, even when food has really baked on, and they can go in the dishwasher. Because I do most of my baking with low-calorie cooking spray rather than oil, things are more prone to stick to the tray.

Oven dishes: I love my vintage-looking enamel rectangular oven dishes. I also have a really useful ovenproof glass dish, which I admit doesn't look as pretty for presentation, but is very handy, washable, and has a lid, so it's good for storing leftovers in the refrigerator as well.

Baking parchment: Cooking without much oil or fat does leave things prone to sticking, so baking parchment is invaluable. If you prefer, you can use washable silicone baking mats.

Loaf tin: A few recipes in this book require a loaf tin, and I use mine a lot.

Loaf tin liners: These are brilliant for enabling you to lift a cake or loaf from the tin without it sticking.

Garlic press: I find it much easier to use this than to chop garlic cloves.

Colander: For draining pasta, rice and vegetables.

Zester: I use citrus zest a lot to add flavour to meals and when baking, and it tends to be easier to use a zester than a grater. Always zest the fruit before juicing it though.

Juicer: To squeeze the juice out of all those lovely lemons, limes and oranges for flavouring sauces, salads and cakes.

Measuring spoons: Most of the recipes in this book use measuring spoons as a guide to get the balance of flavours right. It makes sense to have an accurate and consistent measure, as different cutlery can really vary in volume.

Good-quality sharp knife: Being able to chop efficiently is really important when you are doing lots of cooking! Twenty years ago I invested in two really good-quality knives – a cook's knife and a paring knife – and they are still all I use.

Knife sharpener: It's important to keep knives sharp, as it makes preparing food so much easier. I have a ceramic knife sharpener.

Chopping boards: Having separate, dedicated boards for meats and fruit/vegetables prevents cross-contamination. You can buy sets or just get chopping boards in different colours for quick identification.

Rubber spatula: For scraping sauces out of pans, hummus out of the food processor bowl and cake batters into tins.

Tongs: Handy for serving up food or turning hot food in a pan.

Whisk: For fluffy egg whites.

Measuring jug: For making sure the volume of liquid you are adding to dishes is correct according to the recipe.

Ramekins: Handy for baked oats, crumble, or mixing up salad dressings.

Steamer: I have a cheap bamboo steamer that sits on top of a saucepan. It's a great way to cook vegetables, minimizing nutrient loss.

Accurate kitchen scales: Important for getting the measurements right in recipes.

Empty jam jars: I clean out empty jam jars and save them for storing my spice mixes or chia seed jam, making overnight oats or keeping leftover pasta sauce in the refrigerator – so handy!

APPLIANCES

Slow cooker: My grandma bought me my first slow cooker when I was at university, and it is still going strong 22 years later. I love using a slow cooker for occasions where you just want to come home to a hot meal. They are good value, a safe way to leave food unattended while it's cooking, and there are so many recipes you can try in them – and loads in this book – from curries and casseroles to cakes and bread, or even overnight breakfasts.

Hand blender: A cheap model does the job. I've had a basic supermarket version for years and it's ideal for blending soups and sauces.

Mini chopper: A great labour saver when making curries, as you can quickly blend onions, garlic and chilli to save a lot of chopping by hand. Great for dips too.

Food processor: Another great time saver. I didn't have one for years, but now I couldn't live without it. I use it a lot for making dips and blending up sauces, and mine has a grater, which is brilliant for meals that use a lot of grated carrot or red cabbage.

NOTES

Oven: I tested all the recipes in this book using a fan-assisted oven. If you are using a conventional oven, you may need to adjust cooking times or temperatures.

Cooking: There are so many variables with cooking, to do with temperatures, individual cooking ability, utensils and ingredients. Don't worry, most of the recipes in this book won't be ruined by slight changes to these factors.

Calories: The calorie counts stated in each recipe are for a single portion and do not include serving suggestions or side dishes. Calorie calculations can vary, based on precision of measurements, brands of ingredients or the source of nutrition data. The information provided should be used as a guide.

Cooking spray/spray oil: I use low-calorie cooking spray for most of my cooking. It's a great way to cut down on calories and I've always found to it be an effective medium. If you prefer, a spray oil can be used instead.

Chilli: I adore chilli, and I think it adds so much flavour and depth to dishes (even for breakfast – try it). If you aren't a fan of hot food you can easily reduce the amount in these dishes, or even cut it out. The heat levels of chillies can really vary so, if you aren't sure how hot yours are, it's worth exercising caution!

Eggs: I always use free-range eggs and unless otherwise specified I use large eggs.

Meat: Always buy the best you can afford. By using a good butcher you have a great source of knowledge to tap into; they can tailor cuts to your taste, do any filleting and ensure you get a lean cut.

Seasonal eating: Eating vegetables and fruits in season makes sense. In-season produce tastes nicer, is better value and supports local farming. Lots of the recipes in this book allow ingredients to be substituted, to accommodate what is in season.

Nutritional information: Please note, I am not a certified dietitian or nutritionist. This book is a collection of recipes that I eat and enjoy as part of a balanced diet. I hope they will provide you with some ideas and options to try, but everyone is different and this book is not meant to replace any dietary advice from your own qualified professional.

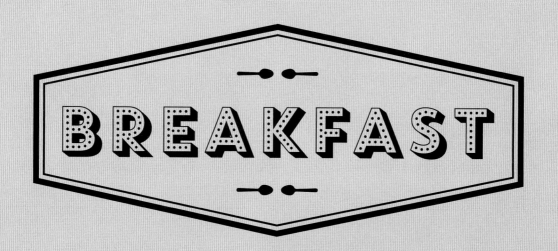

• • • • • • • • • • • • •

Mornings can be a busy time of day, but that's no reason not to kick them off with a good breakfast. It will give you energy and limit mid-morning snacking temptations, and choosing a healthy breakfast is a great motivator to inspire you to keep eating well throughout the day.

One of my favourite breakfasts is baked oats. They are so cakey and delicious that they taste like a real treat. Baking Raspberry & Cinnamon Baked Oats with Toasted Almond Topping first thing in the morning always sends the most delicious smells wafting through the house.

There's nothing like waking up to a breakfast that is ready to go, especially something warming and filling. That is why I love to use the slow cooker to put Slow-cooker Creamy Overnight Porridge on the night before, leaving it to simmer gently overnight and provide a hot, creamy breakfast first thing. Overnight oats are also a great choice to prepare in advance, perfect for when you need a grab-and-go option that is also satisfying and delicious.

Sometimes you just need something simple and sweet to go with your porridge or spread on a piece of toast, so I've included a recipe for my homemade Easy Chia Seed Summer Fruit Jam, which is much lower in sugar than most bought jams and delicious and versatile too.

With a bit more time at the weekend, there's the chance to cook something a bit more indulgent, such as a filling Brunch Hash with runny, golden-yolked eggs, or a hot, cheesy Chilli Bacon Breakfast Quesadilla. These always make me happy and hit the spot every time.

• • • • • • • • • • • • •

RASPBERRY & CINNAMON BAKED OATS

WITH TOASTED ALMOND TOPPING

Such a dreamy and satisfying breakfast: warmly scented cinnamon and raspberries in cakey-textured oats, with a crunchy, golden almond topping. Serve with fat-free yogurt and sweet fresh berries for the perfect combination.

CALORIES PER SERVING: 351

60g (2¼oz) porridge oats
2 teaspoons baking powder
½ teaspoon ground cinnamon
1 tablespoon stevia sweetener
1 egg
4 tablespoons fat-free Greek yogurt, plus extra to serve
100g (3½oz) fresh or frozen raspberries, plus extra to serve
low-calorie cooking spray
10g (¼oz) flaked almonds
salt

1. Preheat the oven to 200°C/180°C fan (400°F), Gas Mark 6.
2. Mix together the oats, baking powder, cinnamon, sweetener and a small pinch of salt. Crack in the egg and spoon in the yogurt, then mix everything together well.
3. Stir the raspberries through the oat mixture. Prepare 2 ramekins by spraying with low-calorie cooking spray, then divide the mixture evenly between the ramekins.
4. Sprinkle the flaked almonds evenly over the top, spray with cooking spray, then place on the middle shelf of the oven and cook for 35 minutes.
5. Serve the baked oats straightaway, still in their ramekins, with the crunchy almonds on top, with fresh raspberries and fat-free yogurt on the side.

NOTE These are also delicious made with blueberries, blackberries or frozen mixed berries, or, for a change, replace the cinnamon with vanilla extract. To save on time in the morning, you can make up the dry mix (oats, baking powder, cinnamon, sweetener and salt) in advance. Store in a jam jar, then just stir in the wet ingredients when you are ready to bake.

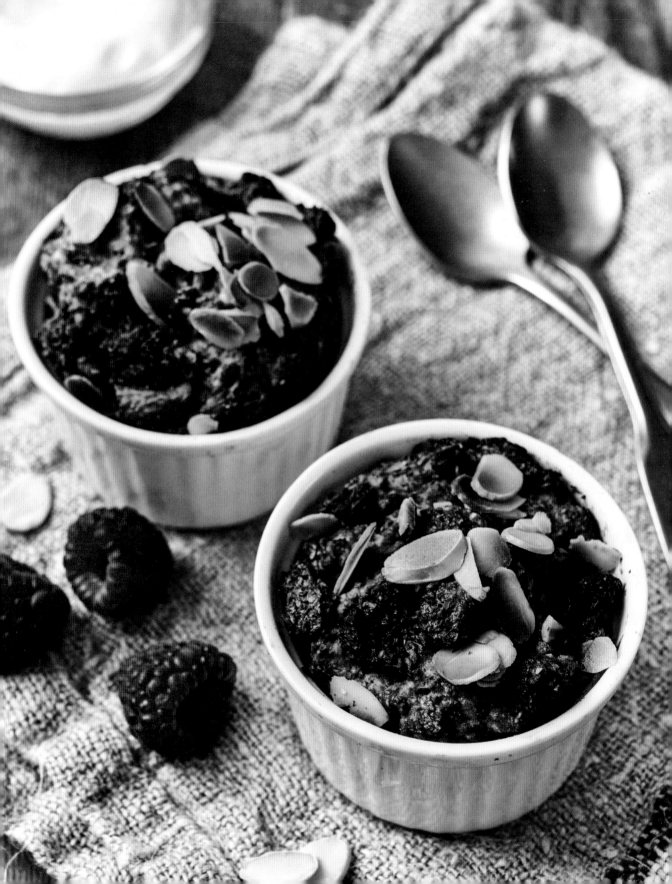

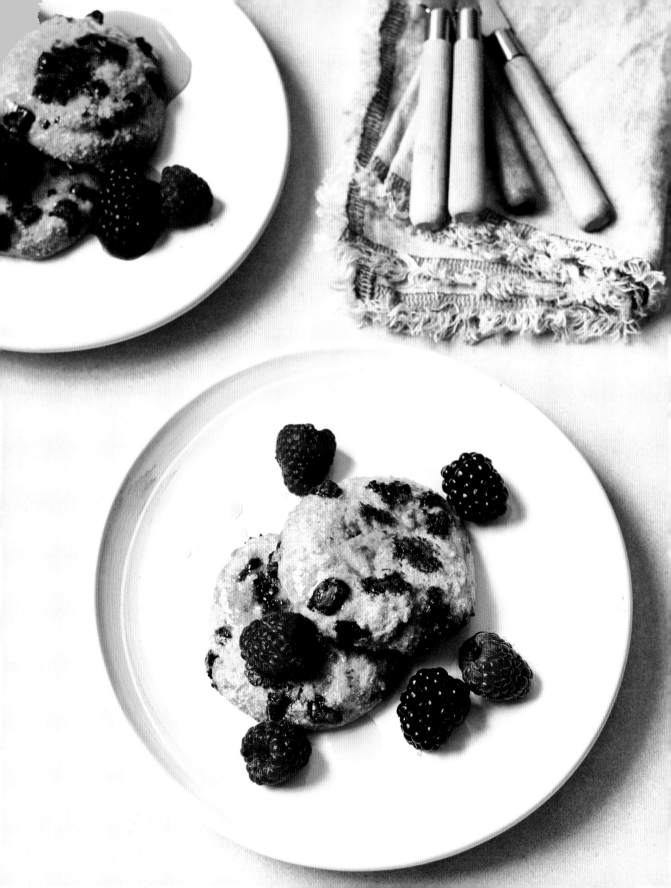

CHOCOLATE, HAZELNUT & OAT OVEN-BAKED PANCAKES

With warm, softly melting chocolate chips and a rich hazelnut taste, these pancakes are crisp on the outside and fluffy in the middle. Baking them means they cook perfectly each time, and they are so simple to make. I love these served with fresh, sweet strawberries and a little drizzle of maple syrup.

CALORIES PER SERVING: 368

60g (2¼oz) oats
12 whole hazelnuts
1 teaspoon baking powder
1 egg
80g (2¾oz) fat-free Greek yogurt
1 teaspoon vanilla extract
25g (1oz) milk chocolate chips
low-calorie cooking spray
salt

TO SERVE
fresh berries of your choice
maple syrup

1. Preheat the oven to 200°C/180°C fan (400°F), Gas Mark 6.
2. In a mini chopper, blend together the oats, hazelnuts, baking powder, egg, Greek yogurt, vanilla extract and a pinch of salt until the oats and nuts are broken down to a textured batter.
3. Stir in the chocolate chips.
4. Line a baking tray with baking parchment, spray it with low-calorie cooking spray and use a tablespoon to dollop the mixture into 4 pancakes. Make sure to space them out over the tray, so they don't stick together.
5. Spray the tops with cooking spray and bake on the top shelf of the oven for 10 minutes.
6. After 10 minutes, use a spatula to flip the pancakes and bake for another 5 minutes. When you remove them from the oven they should be golden brown and a little crisp on the outside, but fluffy on the inside.
7. Serve with fresh berries of your choice and a small drizzle of maple syrup.

NOTE These can be easily adapted with different flavours: try a pinch of ground cinnamon, some finely grated orange zest or replace the chocolate chips with blueberries.

SLOW-COOKER CREAMY OVERNIGHT PORRIDGE

Spending just 5 minutes prepping before you go to bed will allow you to wake up to a bowl of perfect, creamy, warming porridge. This is ideal for those busy mornings when you just need something that is ready to go. The slow cooking overnight gives the oats an unbeatable creamy texture. It's important to use jumbo porridge oats for this, as due to the long cooking time other types of oats are likely to go too mushy. I think they always make the best porridge anyway. A combination of milk and water will give the oats a well-balanced consistency and flavour, without being too stodgy. Simply serve with your favourite toppings, such as sliced banana, a handful of fresh blueberries, a drizzle of honey or maple syrup, a sprinkling of nuts or some homemade Easy Chia Seed Summer Fruit Jam (see opposite).

CALORIES PER SERVING: 185

low-calorie cooking spray
240g (8½oz) jumbo porridge oats
500ml (18fl oz) semi-skimmed milk
1.2 litres (2 pints) water
salt

1. Spray the slow-cooker bowl with low-calorie cooking spray, then add the oats, milk, measured water and a pinch of salt. Give everything a stir, place the lid on and turn the dial to low.
2. Cook on low for 8 hours.
3. When ready to serve, remove the lid, give everything a good stir to break up any crusty parts that have formed around the side, and serve with your favourite toppings.

NOTE Slow cookers can vary both in size and temperature, which can affect the consistency of the porridge. If it seems too thick, you can loosen it up with a splash of milk. If you have any left over, just cover it and put it in the refrigerator for the next day. You can then microwave it to warm it through, and again just loosen it up with a little extra milk if the consistency has become a little jelly-like.

EASY CHIA SEED SUMMER FRUIT JAM

This jam can be whipped up in just 10 minutes and is thickened with nutrient-rich chia seeds rather than added sugar. It's perfect on top of porridge, pancakes, served with yogurt or granola, or even just spread on toast. My children love it on freshly baked Scrumptious No-added-sugar Teabread (see page 202). It will last for 1 week in the refrigerator.

CALORIES PER SERVING: 23

250g (9oz) frozen summer fruit mix
1 teaspoon vanilla extract
1 tablespoon honey
2 tablespoons chia seeds

1. In a small saucepan, warm the fruit over a low heat until soft, then add the vanilla extract and honey.
2. Bring up to a simmer, then cook gently for 3–4 minutes.
3. Using a potato masher, mash the fruit up as much as you can.
4. Stir in the chia seeds, then transfer to a 250ml (9fl oz) jam jar (or an equivalent-sized Tupperware container).
5. Allow to cool, stir again, then store in the refrigerator.

NOTE I have used 1 tablespoon of honey as the summer fruit mix can be quite tart. You can try this recipe out with all sorts of different berries though. Some – such as strawberries – are naturally sweeter, so you may not need the honey at all, or just start with 1 teaspoon of honey and adjust to taste.

REFRESHING PASSION FRUIT & RASPBERRY OVERNIGHT OATS

Overnight oats are a fantastic make-ahead breakfast for an easy start to the day. I love the combination of exotic passion fruit and flavoursome raspberries. I prefer to use frozen raspberries – as they defrost overnight, the juice infuses into the yogurt and oats, creating a creamy, spoonable consistency. Both passion fruit and raspberries can vary greatly in sweetness, so you may find that you wish to add a drizzle of honey or maple syrup to sweeten things if the ones you use are very tart.

CALORIES PER SERVING: 296

40g (1½oz) porridge oats
150g (5½oz) fat-free Greek yogurt
40g (1½oz) frozen raspberries
2 passion fruit

1. The night before you want the oats, choose a glass jar with a lid. Sprinkle one-third of the oats into the bottom, cover with one-third of the yogurt, then one-third of the raspberries.
2. Cut 1 passion fruit in half, and scoop the pulp out of one-half to go over the raspberries.
3. Repeat the layering of the oats, yogurt, raspberries and passion fruit twice more, but for the very top layer use the pulp of 1 whole passion fruit.
4. Place the lid on the jar and pop in the refrigerator ready for the morning.

NOTE Cleaned-out jam jars are the perfect container for overnight oats, and they look so pretty made this way! If you want something more transportable for breakfast on-the-go, then use a sealed, watertight container. Experiment with different types of fruit, or flavoured yogurts, for variety.

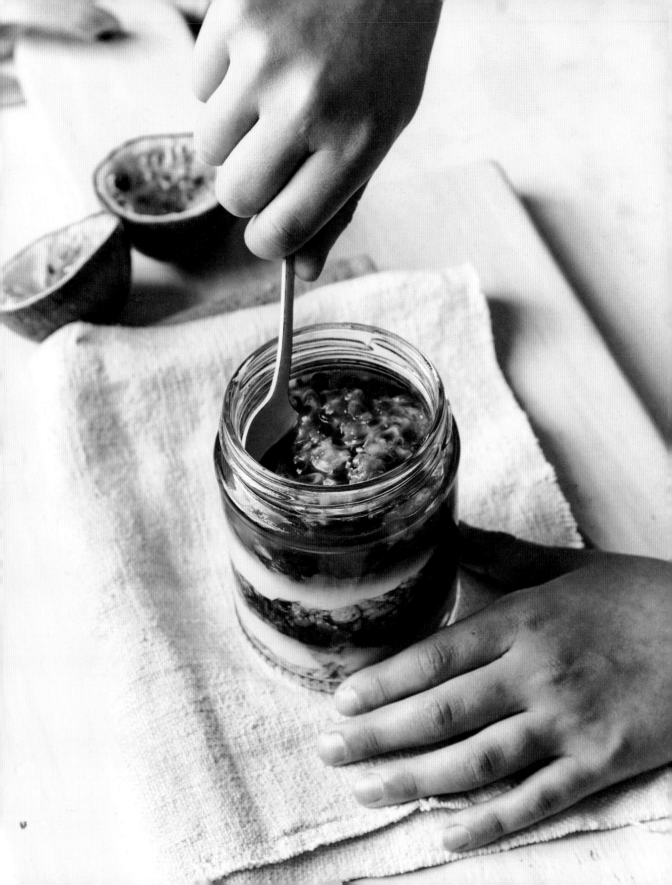

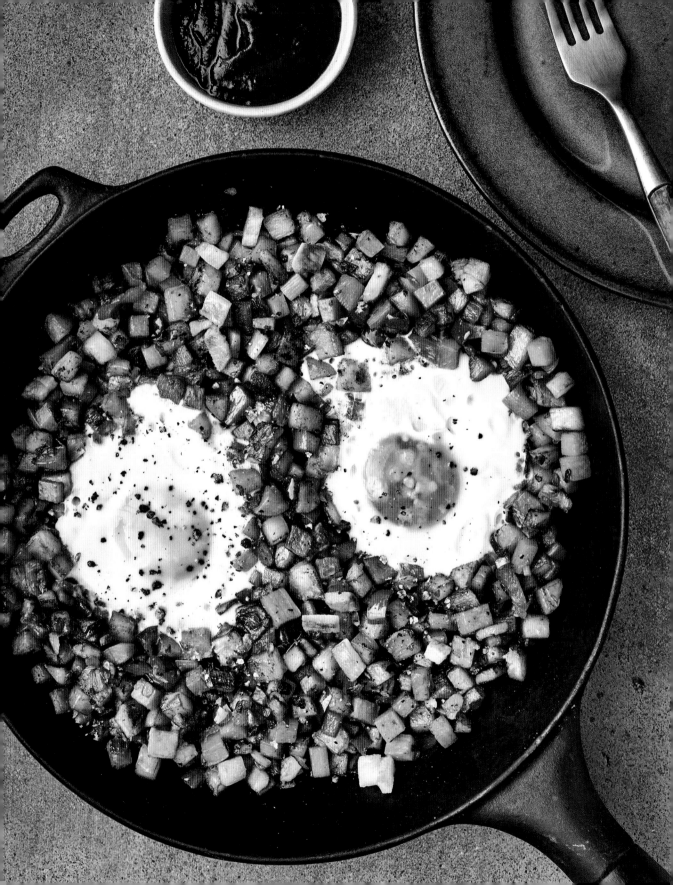

BRUNCH HASH

A hearty one-pan dish, this is my go-to Saturday brunch, which I usually squeeze in after the dog walk and before the kids' swimming lessons to keep us fuelled for a busy day! It has the filling power of a full cooked breakfast, but the ease of everything being cooked in one pan. This is great on its own, but sometimes I like to serve it with baked beans on the side.

CALORIES PER SERVING: 360

low-calorie cooking spray

1 medium white potato (about 200g / 7oz), peeled and chopped into smallish cubes

1 red onion, finely chopped

2 smoked back bacon rashers, fat removed, finely chopped

1 medium sweet potato (about 200g / 7oz), peeled and chopped into smallish cubes

½ red pepper, deseeded and chopped intro smallish cubes

2 eggs

salt and pepper

sauce of your choice (brown sauce or chilli sauce work perfectly), to serve

1. Spray a sauté pan with low-calorie cooking spray, place over a high heat and tip in the white potato. Stir-fry for 5 minutes, until it is starting to lightly brown on the outside.

2. Add in the onion and bacon, reduce the heat slightly and stir-fry for 5 more minutes.

3. Add the sweet potato and pepper to the pan, spray the top with a little more cooking spray and cook over a medium heat for 20 minutes, stirring regularly.

4. Push aside the vegetables with a wooden spoon to create 2 small hollows in the hash. Crack the eggs into these.

5. Season everything with salt and pepper, place a lid on the pan and allow the eggs to fry for 4 minutes: you want the whites to be cooked through on the top and the yolks to still be runny.

6. Serve immediately with your favourite sauce.

NOTE Make this vegetarian by leaving out the bacon and add in any other breakfast favourites you fancy, such as mushrooms and tomatoes. Torn-up mozzarella also works well in this – just add it at the same time as the eggs.

CHEDDAR & ONION BAKED IRISH BOXTY

Boxty is a traditional Irish pancake made of mashed and grated potatoes. This baked version is crisp on the outside and soft and creamy in the middle. It can be served fresh from the oven on its own, with a fried egg or beans, or as part of a hearty full Irish breakfast.

CALORIES PER SERVING: 214

600g (1lb 5oz) floury white potatoes (such as Roosters), peeled
1 onion, finely chopped
low-calorie cooking spray
1 tablespoon semi-skimmed milk
¼ teaspoon salt
2 tablespoons self-raising flour
60g (2¼oz) Cheddar cheese, grated

1. Preheat the oven to 220°C/200°C fan (425°F), Gas Mark 7.
2. Cut half the potatoes into large chunks and boil them in a large saucepan of water for 15 minutes.
3. In a small frying pan, fry the onion gently in low-calorie cooking spray over a low heat while the potatoes cook. Stir every now and again to prevent burning.
4. Meanwhile, grate the remaining potatoes into a sieve placed over a bowl. Use a piece of kitchen paper to press down and squeeze out the liquid from the grated potato.
5. Remove the fried onions from the heat (they should be translucent and lightly browned).
6. Drain the boiled potatoes, leaving them for a minute in the colander, then empty them into a large bowl, add the milk and salt and mash them until smooth.
7. Stir in the grated potato and flour, then the fried onion and the cheese and stir until thoroughly combined.
8. Line a flan or quiche dish with baking parchment, spray it with cooking spray and spoon in the potato mixture.
9. Smooth over the top of the mixture so it is evenly spread, then score the top with a sharp knife to mark the boxty into quarters. Spray the top with cooking spray.
10. Place the dish on the middle shelf of the oven and bake for 35 minutes, until the top is crisped and golden brown.
11. Slice into quarters, ease carefully away from the baking parchment and serve hot from the oven.

NOTE Try adding herbs or spring onions for extra flavour.

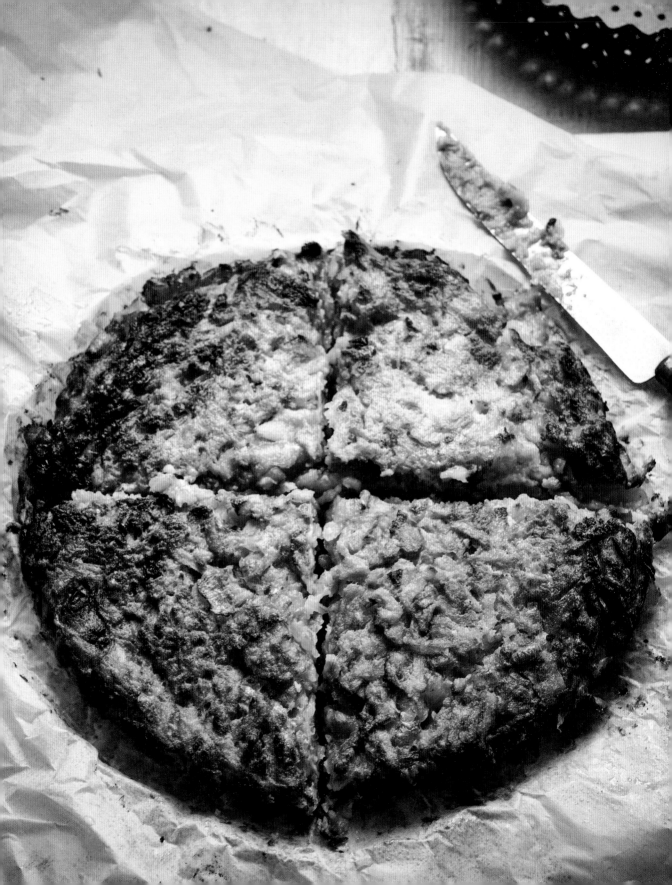

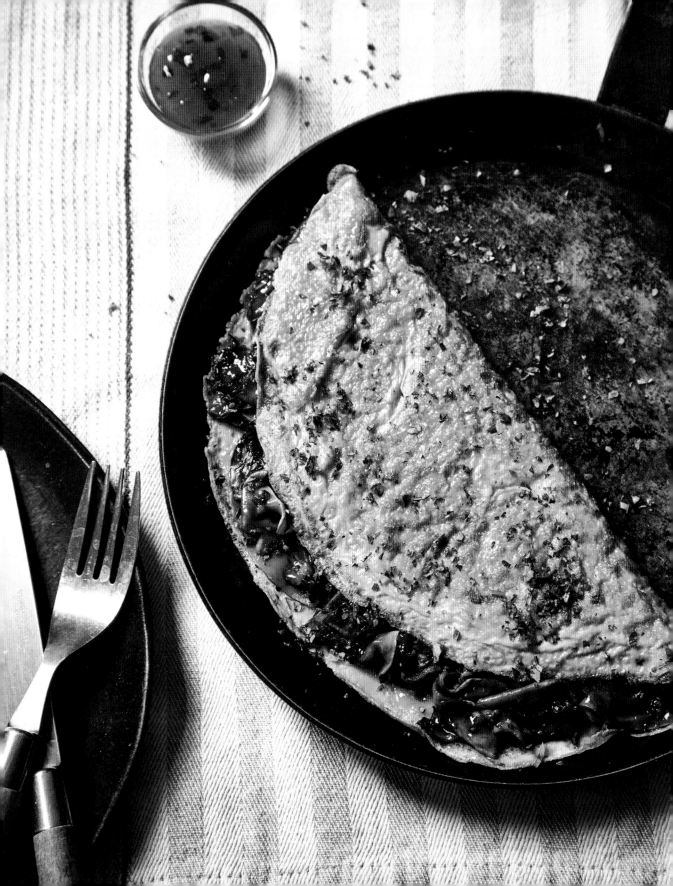

SWEET CHILLI MUSHROOM OMELETTE

Savoury mushrooms and jammy sweet chilli fried together are perfect in a hot, golden, fluffy omelette. When buying eggs, look for the best you can afford, as good-quality, fresh, free-range eggs always make the best omelettes.

CALORIES PER SERVING: 275

1 large flat mushroom, sliced as finely as possible
low-calorie cooking spray
1 tablespoon sweet chilli sauce
3 eggs
salt and pepper
leaves from a few parsley sprigs, finely chopped, to serve

1. Fry the mushroom slices over a high heat in low-calorie cooking spray for 2–3 minutes, then stir in the sweet chilli sauce and remove from the heat.
2. Beat the eggs together thoroughly and add a few grinds of salt and pepper.
3. Spray a medium-sized nonstick frying pan with cooking spray, place over a high heat and pour in the egg.
4. Reduce the heat slightly, and once the egg is starting to set around the edges of the pan, use a wooden spatula to bring the cooked edges of the omelette into the middle of the pan. Then tilt the pan to swirl the runny, uncooked egg to the edges, to cover the bottom of the pan.
5. Keep the heat low and allow the egg to cook through. When it's cooked you won't be able to see any liquid egg remaining on the top.
6. Spoon the mushroom and sweet chilli mixture over one half of the omelette, then fold the other half over the top.
7. Slide the omelette on to a plate and serve immediately with the parsley sprinkled over the top.

NOTE A good, nonstick frying pan will ensure the omelette is a success.

CHILLI BACON BREAKFAST QUESADILLA

Years ago, I used to love grabbing an egg and melted cheese toasted English muffin on my way into work, and this breakfast quesadilla reminds me of that. With its oozing cheesey middle, it feels quite indulgent, but it is also quick and easy to make at home. It's simple to wrap up and take with you for breakfast on the go, limiting those impromptu stops at the local coffee shop...

CALORIES PER SERVING: 475

---

2 lean smoked bacon medallions, finely sliced

2 eggs

low-calorie cooking spray

30g (1oz) Cheddar cheese, grated

1 medium-sized low-fat tortilla wrap

1 teaspoon hot chilli sauce

salt and pepper

1. Fry the sliced bacon in a dry frying pan for a couple of minutes until cooked through. Set aside.
2. Beat the eggs in a bowl and season with salt and pepper.
3. Choose a nonstick frying pan that is a similar size to the wrap you are using (if it's a lot bigger, the egg will spread too much). Spray the pan with low-calorie cooking spray, place over a high heat and pour in the beaten egg.
4. Sprinkle about one-third of the grated cheese over the egg and cook for about a minute, until the egg is nearly cooked through but still a little wet on the top.
5. Place the wrap over the egg and gently press down. Cook for another minute until you can easily slide a spatula under the egg. Flip the tortilla and egg over so that it's tortilla side-down in the pan.
6. Sprinkle the rest of the cheese and the bacon over the egg. Drizzle the chilli sauce over everything.
7. Use the spatula to fold the wrap in half, gently pressing down on it to help it hold its shape.
8. Lift the quesadilla from the pan to a plate and use a sharp knife to cut it in half. Serve immediately.

NOTE You can replace the chilli sauce with brown sauce or tomato ketchup if you prefer, and, for a vegetarian option, replace the bacon with fried mushrooms, cherry tomatoes or fried onions.

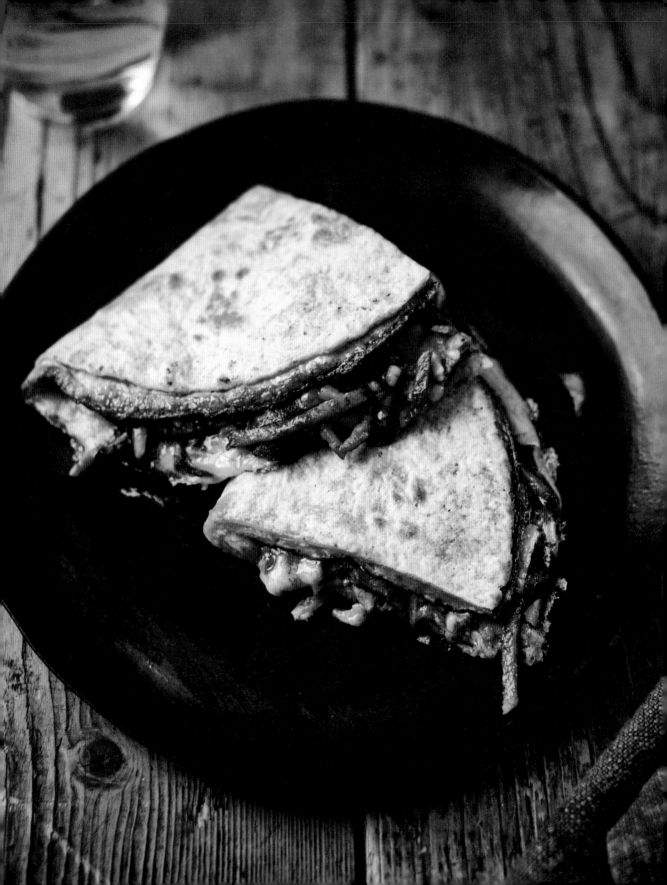

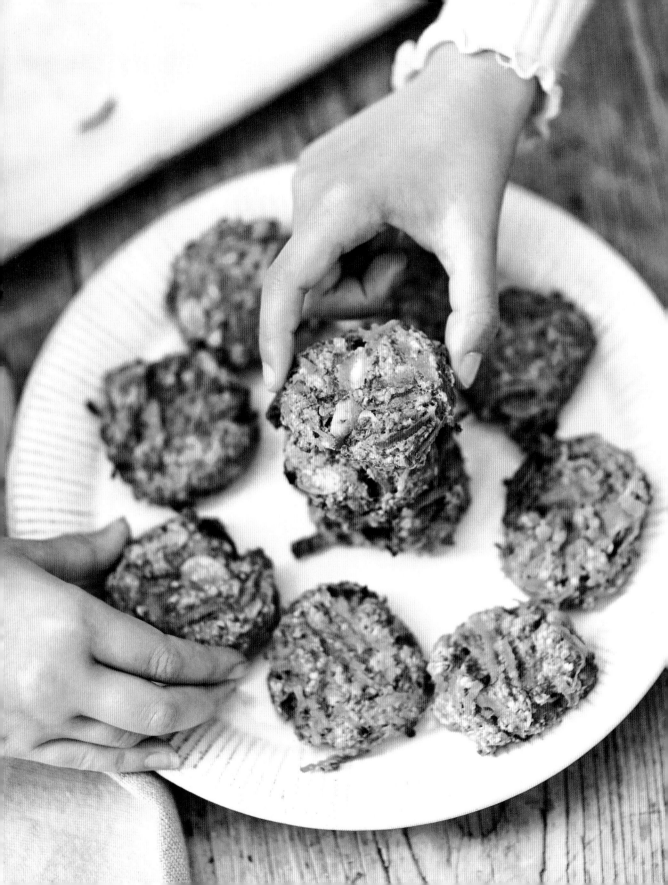

NUTTY GOLDEN CARROT & ORANGE BREAKFAST COOKIES

These make the perfect grab-and-go breakfast. The smell of them baking first thing in the morning is irresistible and they are delicious both warm and cold. Full of fibre, and with no added sugar, they also make a great healthy snack at any time of day.

CALORIES PER COOKIE: 97

80g (2³/₄oz) porridge oats
60g (2¹/₄oz) wholemeal flour
1 teaspoon baking powder
¼ teaspoon salt
20g (³/₄oz) walnuts, chopped
25g (1oz) flaked almonds
2 tablespoons chia seeds
1 egg
1 teaspoon vanilla extract
finely grated zest and juice
    of 1 orange
1 carrot (about 100g / 3¹/₂oz),
    peeled and grated
low-calorie cooking spray

1. Preheat the oven to 220°C/200°C fan (425°F), Gas Mark 7.
2. Mix together the oats, flour, baking powder, salt, walnuts, almonds and chia seeds.
3. Make a well in the middle and add the egg, vanilla extract, orange zest and juice.
4. Stir everything together, then add the grated carrot. Mix well to combine everything thoroughly.
5. Line a large baking tray with baking parchment and spray with a little low-calorie cooking spray.
6. Form the mixture into 12 even-sized balls using your hands. Place these on the baking tray, then use a fork to flatten each one. Spray the tops with a little more cooking spray.
7. Bake in the oven for 12–15 minutes. They should be golden brown and cooked through to the middle.

NOTE The nuts can easily be swapped for your favourites – try hazelnuts, pistachios or macadamia nuts. Or replace the nuts with seeds, such as sunflower seeds or pumpkin seeds. You can prepare the dry mix in advance and store it in an airtight container, ready to add the egg, vanilla, orange and carrot when you are ready to bake the cookies.

QUICK & EASY
MIDWEEK MEALS

• • • • • • • • • • • • • •

I have a few firm favourite recipes that I return to again and again when I need something that's quick to cook. They're winners not only because they're delicious, but because I usually have the ingredients in, or they only require a speedy trolley-dash through the supermarket.

After a long day at work, or a busy weekend day out, it's reassuring to know that I have healthy options to turn to that take little time and effort. Having recipes like these up my sleeve is a great way to still eat healthily during a busy week.

If I have some leftover roast chicken from the weekend, I'll often knock up a Thai Chicken Noodle Soup; I particularly love it on a cold winter's evening next to a roaring fire. When my refrigerator is looking a little bare, pulling together a Lightning-quick Tuna, Chilli & Cannellini Bean Linguine is the ideal solution, as it mainly uses canned and dried ingredients and can be ready to eat in 15 minutes. There are times when I'll have an impromptu night in with friends, and that's when I turn to Jalapeño & Roasted Red Pepper Mac'n'cheese. It's real comfort food, but with very little work and few ingredients.

If you need an extra time-saver, don't hesitate to use jars of pre-chopped chilli, ginger and garlic if they keep life simple – the food will still taste great!

• • • • • • • • • • • • • •

PORTOBELLO PIZZAS

Pizzas are a popular treat in my house, and substituting Portobello mushrooms for traditional dough pizza bases gives a healthy twist on a familiar favourite. With little preparation time needed and being quick to cook too, these make a fantastic speedy meal. Serve with a rocket salad.

CALORIES PER SERVING: 178

---

4 Portobello mushrooms
low-calorie cooking spray
4 teaspoons tomato purée
½ teaspoon garlic granules
60g (2¼oz) Cheddar cheese, grated
4 cherry tomatoes, quartered
1 teaspoon dried oregano
salt and pepper
rocket leaves, to serve

1. Preheat the oven to 200°C/180°C fan (400°F), Gas Mark 6.
2. Place the mushrooms with the stalks facing upwards on a baking tray and trim away the stalks.
3. Spray each mushroom with low-calorie cooking spray and season with salt and pepper. Put the mushrooms in the oven to bake for 10 minutes.
4. When the mushrooms come out of the oven, tip out any excess liquid that has pooled inside them.
5. Put a teaspoon of tomato purée in each mushroom and spread it around, then sprinkle a pinch of garlic granules over each one. Divide the cheese equally between the 4 mushrooms.
6. Top each mushroom with a quartered cherry tomato, then sprinkle with dried oregano.
7. Bake the mushrooms for another 10 minutes until the cheese is melted and golden.
8. Serve with a rocket salad.

NOTE If you have a batch of Make-ahead Marinara Sauce in the refrigerator (see page 214), it makes a great replacement for the tomato purée. Add whatever pizza toppings you like: pepperoni, jalapeños, or even ham and pineapple.

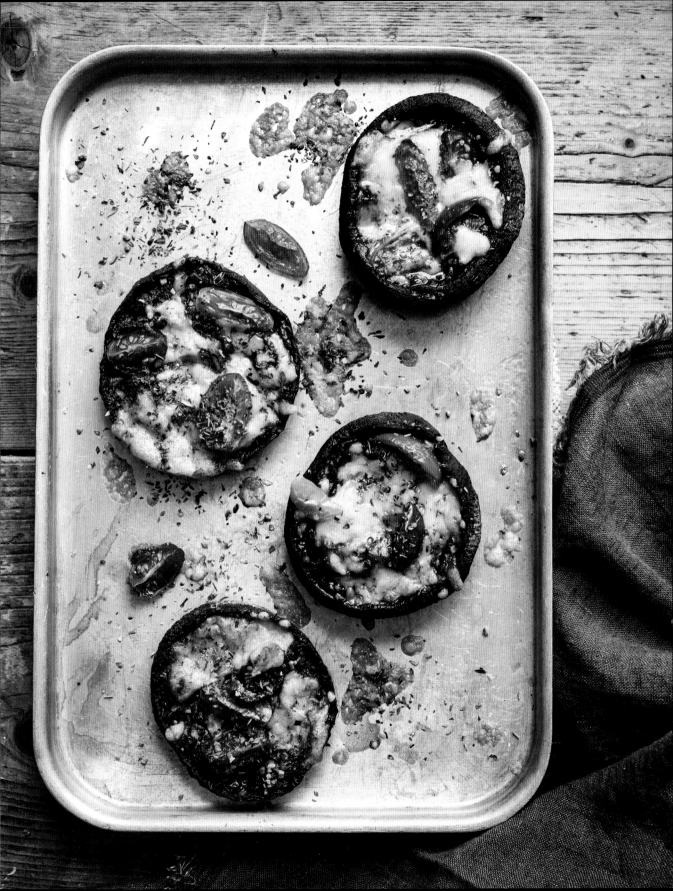

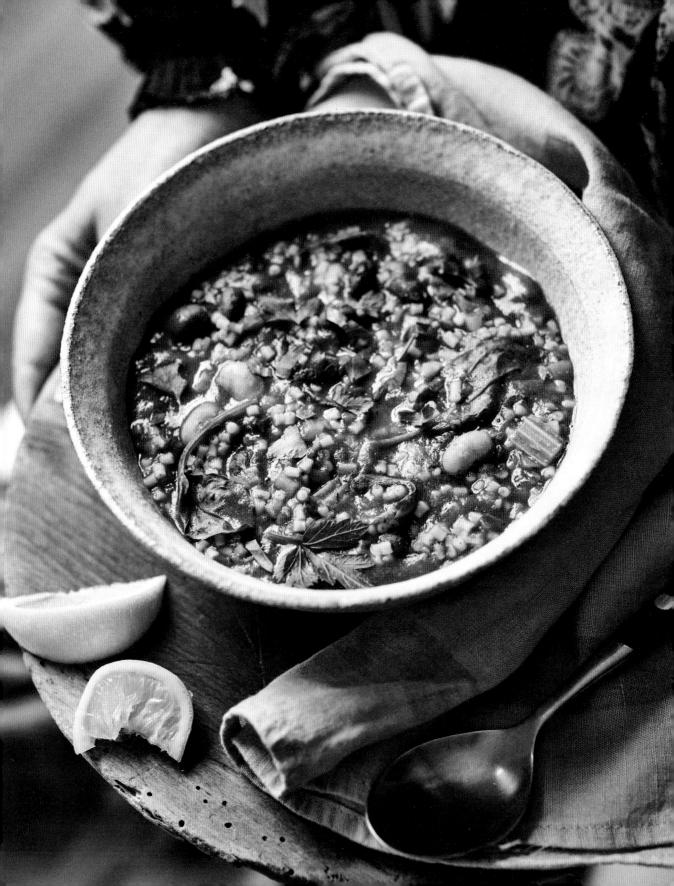

PASTA E FAGIOLI

This is a favourite for me if I'm making lunch for friends or family, because the pan can go straight on the table for everyone to help themselves. It's a comforting, hearty and filling dish, full of classic Italian flavours.

CALORIES PER SERVING: 336

1 large onion, finely chopped

2 celery sticks, finely chopped

2 carrots, peeled and very finely chopped

low-calorie cooking spray

2 garlic cloves, crushed

2 rosemary sprigs, stalks removed, leaves finely chopped

1 teaspoon dried oregano

250g (9oz) tomato passata

1 litre (1¾ pints) vegetable stock

400g (14oz) can borlotti beans, drained and rinsed

400g (14oz) can cannellini beans, drained and rinsed

125g (4½oz) small dried pasta shapes or dried macaroni

30g (1oz) spinach, roughly chopped

juice of ½ lemon

salt and pepper

handful of parsley leaves, to serve

1. Fry the onion, celery and carrots gently in low-calorie cooking spray for about 10 minutes, until softened.
2. Stir in the garlic, rosemary and oregano, and stir-fry for 30 seconds.
3. Pour in the passata and stock and bring up to a rapid simmer.
4. Add both cans of beans and continue to simmer gently for 10 minutes.
5. Remove about one-third of the soup from the pan and blend it using a hand blender. Return the blended soup to the pan.
6. Tip the pasta into the pan, season with salt and pepper, and simmer gently for 20 minutes, until the pasta is cooked through.
7. Stir through the spinach, squeeze in the lemon juice, taste to check the seasoning and serve with the parsley scattered over the top.

NOTE You could also use butter beans or kidney beans in this dish, or replace the spinach with chopped kale. Some freshly grated Parmesan is delicious sprinkled over the top.

CREAMY MUSHROOM, ROSEMARY & PEA ORZOTTO

I like making risotto-style one-pot dishes using orzo, as it doesn't involve the constant stirring needed for a risotto made with rice and it cooks much more quickly, but still has a lovely texture and creamy consistency. Serve with a simple spinach or rocket salad.

CALORIES PER SERVING: 375

low-calorie cooking spray
1 onion, finely chopped
250g (9oz) chestnut mushrooms, sliced
3 garlic cloves, crushed
1 tablespoon very finely chopped rosemary leaves, plus extra to serve
300g (10½oz) dried orzo pasta
50ml (2fl oz) white wine
1 litre (1¾ pints) vegetable stock
150g (5½oz) frozen peas
2 tablespoons half-fat crème fraîche
salt and pepper

1. Spray a sauté pan with low-calorie cooking spray, place over a medium heat and add the onion and mushrooms. Fry for 10 minutes, stirring occasionally.
2. Add the garlic and rosemary and stir-fry for 30 seconds, then tip in the orzo and stir-fry for another minute.
3. Increase the heat to high, pour in the wine, stir well, then pour in 700ml (1¼ pints) of the stock.
4. Keep at a rapid simmer for 15 minutes, stirring occasionally to make sure the orzo doesn't stick to the bottom of the pan. After 15 minutes, add the frozen peas and stir through, then top up with the remaining stock.
5. Simmer for another 5 minutes, stirring continuously until the orzo is tender. Season with salt and pepper and stir in the crème fraîche.
6. Serve immediately with a little more chopped rosemary scattered over the top.

NOTE If you'd like to add meat to this, smoked bacon pieces fried with the onions and mushrooms make a tasty addition.

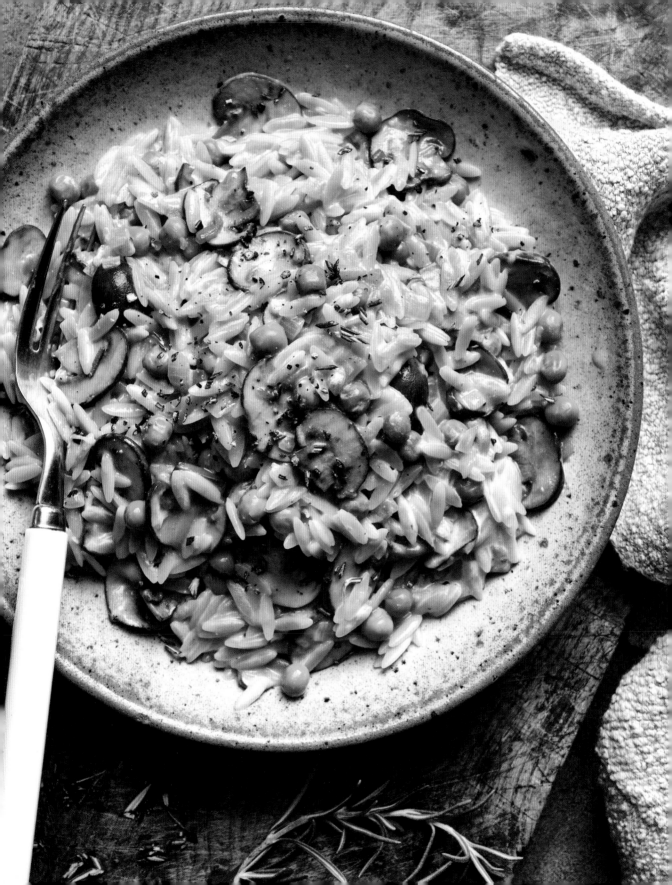

JALAPEÑO & ROASTED RED PEPPER MAC'N'CHEESE

Cooking the macaroni in milk bestows a lovely, creamy texture before the cheese is even added, making it taste much more indulgent than it is.

CALORIES PER SERVING: 451

300g (10½oz) dried macaroni
250ml (9fl oz) semi-skimmed milk
500ml (18fl oz) water
1 teaspoon garlic granules
1 teaspoon onion granules
small handful of pickled jalapeños (about 40g / 1½oz), finely chopped
2 roasted red peppers in brine (about 160g / 5¾oz), drained and finely sliced
90g (3¼oz) Cheddar cheese, grated
¼ teaspoon smoked paprika
salt and pepper

FOR THE CHERRY TOMATO SALAD

500g (1lb 2oz) cherry tomatoes, halved
½ red onion, finely chopped
2 tablespoons red wine vinegar
1 teaspoon dried oregano
freshly ground salt

1. Place the macaroni in a saucepan and cover with the milk and measured water. Add in the garlic and onion granules. Place a lid on the pan and bring up to the boil.
2. Once boiling, remove the lid and reduce to a rapid simmer for 12 minutes, stirring occasionally to prevent the macaroni from sticking to the bottom of the pan. After 12 minutes the macaroni should be cooked through and the sauce no longer watery. If the macaroni isn't quite cooked, splash in a little more boiling water and continue to cook, stirring, for another couple of minutes. Preheat the grill to its highest setting.
3. Add the jalapeños, red peppers and two-thirds of the cheese. Season with salt and pepper, then stir everything together.
4. Decant into an ovenproof dish, scatter the remaining cheese evenly over the top, then sprinkle with the smoked paprika.
5. To make the tomato salad, simply mix the halved cherry tomatoes with the onion, vinegar and oregano and season with salt.
6. Place the macaroni dish under the hot grill for 4–5 minutes until the cheese on top is bubbling and starting to brown. Serve immediately with the cherry tomato salad.

NOTE This is an easy dish to scale up if you are feeding more than 4 people. It can also make a great side dish as part of a Mexican or Tex-Mex feast.

LEMONY LEEK LENTILS WITH HALLOUMI

Canned lentils make this a quick and easy meal, which is flavourful, filling and easy to scale up or down depending how many you are cooking for. If you'd like to serve extra vegetables, some grilled asparagus or Tenderstem broccoli go perfectly.

CALORIES PER SERVING: 518

---

1 leek, trimmed, cleaned and very finely chopped

1 garlic clove, crushed

low-calorie cooking spray

2 x 400g (14oz) cans green lentils, drained and rinsed

250ml (9fl oz) vegetable stock

1 tablespoon tomato purée

1 teaspoon Dijon mustard

½ teaspoon dried thyme

juice of ½ lemon

140g (5oz) halloumi, finely sliced

2 large handfuls of baby spinach, roughly chopped

salt and pepper

small handful of parsley leaves, finely chopped, to serve

1. In a sauté pan, fry the leek and the garlic gently in low-calorie cooking spray for 5 minutes.
2. Add the lentils, stock, tomato purée, mustard, thyme and lemon juice. Season to taste with salt and pepper, then stir well and allow to simmer for 12 minutes.
3. Meanwhile, fry the halloumi. Simply put it in a hot nonstick frying pan (no cooking spray needed) and allow to toast for about 2 minutes on each side until it starts to turn golden-brown. Set aside.
4. When the lentils have cooked for 12 minutes, stir the spinach through for another minute or so to wilt it.
5. Spoon the lentils into serving bowls, top with the halloumi and scatter with the parsley before serving.

NOTE This lentil base also works well with fried chicken or salmon fillets instead of halloumi, or some roasted sweet potato cubes. Any leftover halloumi can be chopped and added to a curry, such as the Balti 'Sauce for Everything' Curry (see page 215), or chopped, fried and added to the Warm Spiced Squash & Pumpkin Seed Salad (see page 81).

LIGHTNING-QUICK TUNA, CHILLI & CANNELLINI BEAN LINGUINE

This meal is an absolute star for using storecupboard ingredients to make an easy, quick and nutritious dish. If you fancy some more vegetables alongside, try serving it with a Ribboned Courgette & Zesty Lemon Salad (see page 134).

CALORIES PER SERVING: 417

300g (10½oz) dried linguine

400g (14oz) can cannellini beans, drained and rinsed

200g (7oz) fine green beans, cut into 2cm (¾ inch) pieces

low-calorie cooking spray

2 garlic cloves, crushed

2 × 145g (5¼oz) cans tuna in spring water, drained

juice of ½ lemon

1 teaspoon chilli flakes

large handful of parsley leaves, finely chopped

salt and pepper

1. Put the linguine in a large saucepan of boiling water to start cooking, and set a timer for 10 minutes.

2. When the timer goes off, put the cannellini beans and green beans in to cook with the linguine for another 3 minutes.

3. Heat a frying pan with low-calorie cooking spray and add the garlic. Sizzle for about 30 seconds, then add the tuna, lemon juice and chilli, along with a couple of tablespoons of the water from the linguine pan, and stir-fry for a couple of minutes.

4. Check the linguine is cooked, then drain it along with the cannellini and green beans, and return it all to the large saucepan. Add the tuna mixture with half the parsley. Season well with salt and pepper and mix everything thoroughly.

5. Serve scattered with the rest of the parsley.

NOTE If you're making this for anyone who doesn't like chilli, just serve the chilli flakes alongside the dish to be sprinkled over individual plates. To increase the fibre content, try making this with wholewheat spaghetti.

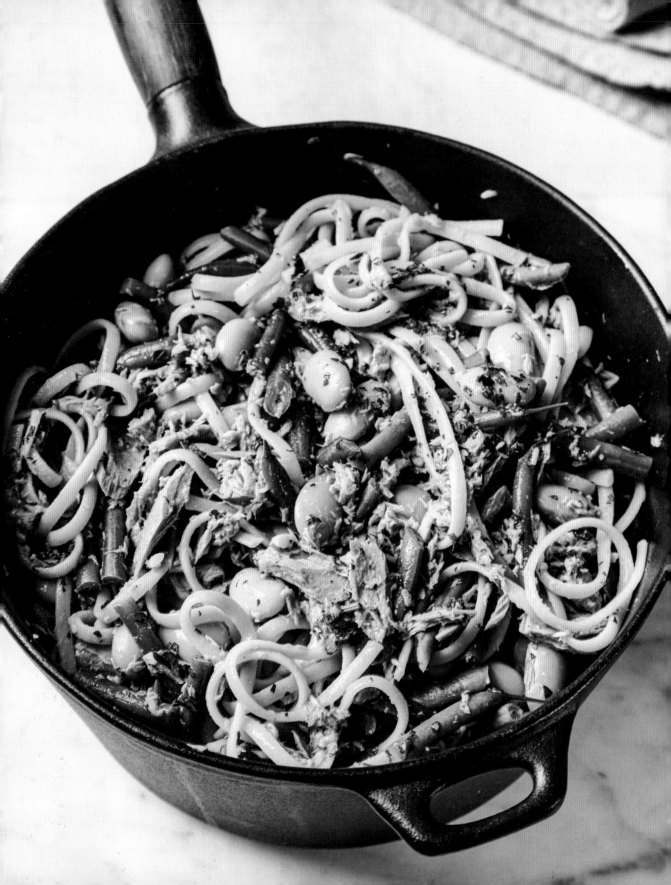

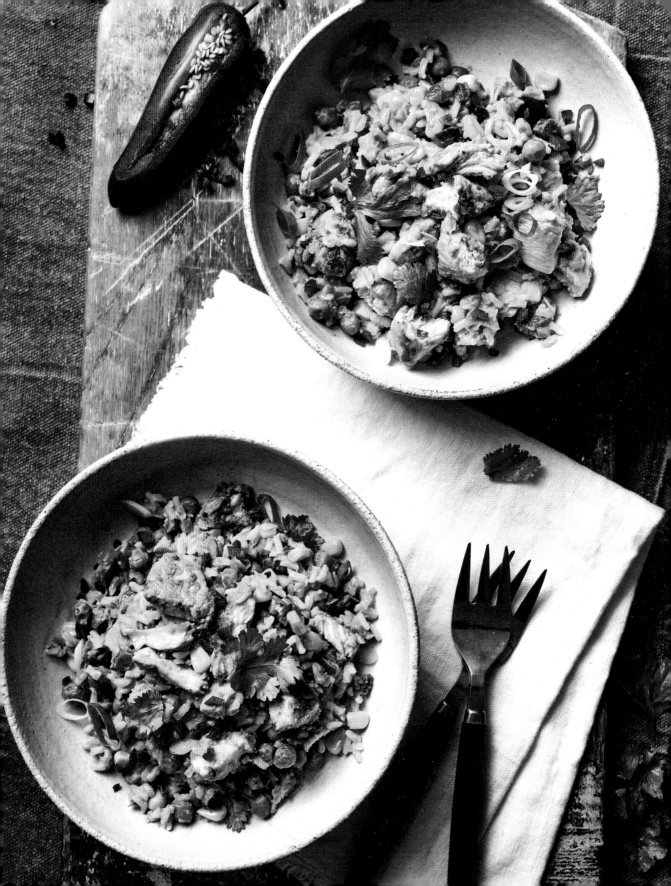

NUTTY CHICKEN SATAY FRIED RICE

A zesty peanut and lime marinade makes this a mouth-watering combination. The nutty brown rice is fantastically satisfying and is a great way to get extra fibre and nutrients. This dish can be pulled together quickly...with delicious results.

CALORIES PER SERVING: 356

2 tablespoons smooth
  peanut butter
2 tablespoons dark soy sauce
finely grated zest and juice
  of 2 unwaxed limes
1 tablespoon fish sauce
2 chicken breasts, chopped
  quite small
200g (7oz) brown rice
4 spring onions, trimmed
  and sliced
1 red pepper, deseeded and
  finely chopped
1 carrot, peeled and finely
  chopped
2 garlic cloves, crushed
1 red chilli, deseeded and
  finely chopped
low-calorie cooking spray
100g (3½oz) frozen peas
100g (3½oz) frozen
  sweetcorn
coriander leaves, to serve

1. Make the marinade by combining the peanut butter, soy sauce, lime zest and juice and fish sauce in a medium-sized bowl. Stir in the chicken and set aside.
2. Put the rice on to cook according to the package instructions (this usually takes about 25 minutes).
3. In a sauté pan or deep frying pan, gently fry the spring onions, pepper, carrot, garlic and chilli in low-calorie cooking spray for 4 minutes.
4. Increase the heat, move the vegetables over to one side of the pan and add the chicken. Once the chicken is sizzling, reduce the heat a little and stir-fry everything gently for 10 minutes.
5. When the brown rice has 5 minutes of cooking time left, add the peas and sweetcorn. When the cooking time is up, drain the rice and vegetables.
6. Add the drained rice and vegetables to the chicken pan and mix everything together thoroughly.
7. Serve sprinkled with coriander leaves.

NOTE You can use up other types of leftover vegetables in this dish, such as celery, leek, broccoli and green beans. For a vegetarian version, marinate cauliflower florets in the satay sauce, to replace the chicken.

THAI CHICKEN NOODLE SOUP

A steaming bowl of this simple but satisfying soup is a year-round winner, with its garlic, chilli, soy and lime elevating the tender chicken. I've used rice stick noodles in this, but you can use any type of noodle you fancy.

CALORIES PER SERVING: 445

2 chicken breasts, cut into strips

low-calorie cooking spray

3 garlic cloves, crushed

2 chillies (ideally 1 red, 1 green), finely chopped

4 spring onions, trimmed and finely sliced

1.4 litres (2½ pints) hot chicken stock

3 tablespoons light soy sauce

1 large carrot, peeled and cut into matchsticks

300g (10½oz) rice stick noodles (see introduction)

150g (5½oz) broccoli florets

50g (1¾oz) fine green beans, halved

1 head of pak choi, trimmed and leaves separated

2 limes, 1 juiced, 1 cut into wedges

handful of coriander leaves, to serve

1. In a large, deep saucepan, fry the chicken in low-calorie cooking spray until no pink is showing on the outside, then add the garlic, chillies and spring onions and stir-fry for a minute.
2. Pour in the hot stock and add the soy sauce and carrots. Simmer for 5 minutes.
3. Now add the noodles, making sure they are submerged, and simmer for 5 minutes.
4. Add the broccoli, green beans and pak choi and simmer for a final 3 minutes.
5. Check that the noodles are cooked through, then stir in the lime juice.
6. Serve immediately, scattered with the coriander and with lime wedges on the side for squeezing over.

NOTE This is a great way to use up homemade Chicken Stock (see page 217) and leftover roast chicken. There are also lots of other vegetables that work well in the soup, such as mushrooms, peppers, sugarsnap peas, beansprouts and spinach.

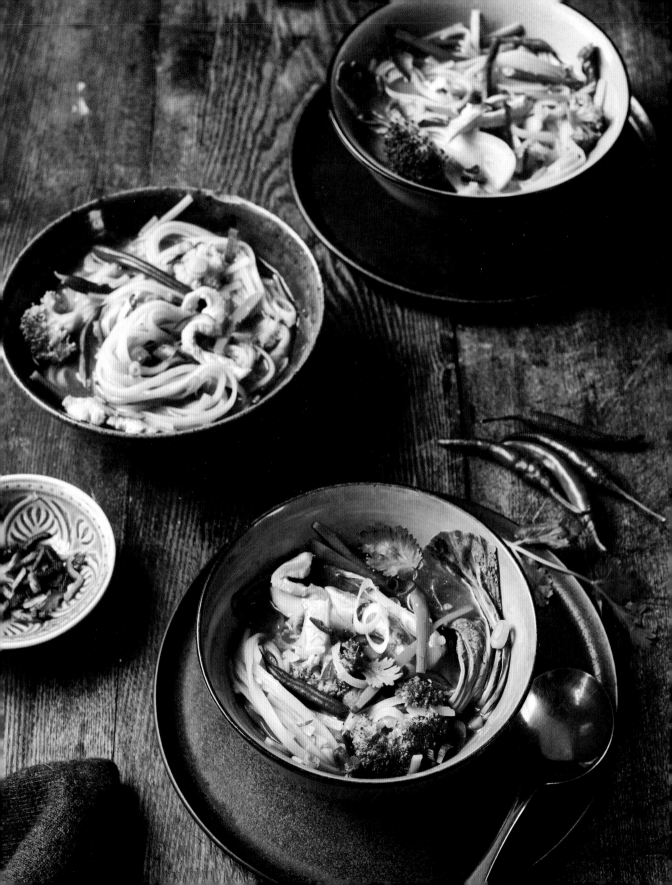

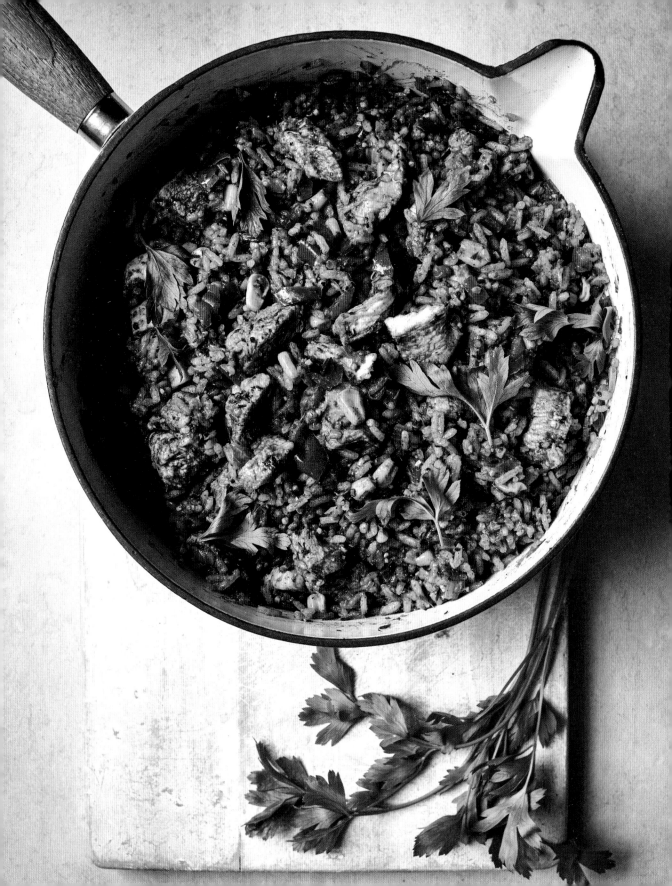

CAJUN CHICKEN RAINBOW RICE

This savoury rice has a deep, spicy flavour and is brilliant for a busy evening. Not only is it quick to make, it's all done in one pan too, so there is minimal washing up. This dish also works cold, so any leftovers can be used for lunch the following day. I'll also make it if I'm planning a picnic, as it gives me a healthy, filling option that's ready to go and easy to share.

CALORIES PER SERVING: 370

1 onion, finely chopped
2 celery sticks, finely chopped
low-calorie cooking spray
2 chicken breasts, chopped small
1 green pepper, deseeded and chopped
1 red pepper, deseeded and chopped
3 tablespoons Cajun Seasoning (see page 213)
250g (9oz) long-grain white rice
500ml (18fl oz) hot chicken stock
100g (3½oz) frozen sweetcorn
pepper
handful of parsley leaves, to serve

1. In a sauté pan with a lid, fry the onion and celery in low-calorie cooking spray for 5 minutes, then add the chicken, peppers and Cajun spice mix. Stir-fry for 5 minutes.
2. Stir in the rice, then pour in the hot stock, add the sweetcorn and mix together. Place the lid on the pan and leave to simmer for 12 minutes.
3. Remove the lid from the pan, fluff the rice through with a fork and simmer for another 2–3 minutes, just to steam off any remaining liquid and ensure that the rice is cooked through.
4. Check the rice is tender, then serve sprinkled with pepper and scattered with the parsley.

NOTE If you want to simplify this even more, you can use frozen pre-cut onion and peppers and pre-diced chicken, to save on preparation time. You could also try using pre-cooked brown rice, adding it at the end of cooking.

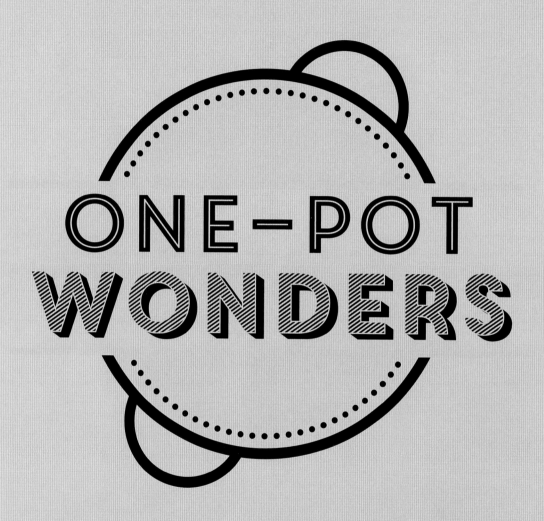

ONE-POT
WONDERS

• • • • • • • • • • • • • •

This has been one of the most popular categories of recipes on my blog. Being able to throw lots of ingredients into one pot and end up with a delicious meal is a joy, plus it's great not to have multiple pans on the go or lots of washing up. A couple of the recipes here are also great for the slow cooker.

One-pot meals are often the best recipes to double up if you want a batch to put in the freezer.

Most of the dishes in this chapter are great for group sharing, whether that's with family over for the weekend, or cooking up a batch of Fiesta Beef for a girls' night in with a movie.

• • • • • • • • • • • • • •

SMOKY MEXICAN BLACK BEAN & SWEET POTATO STEW

I love this rich, dark, smoky and spicy stew. It's full of goodness and is delicious served on its own, or with some rice or quinoa.

CALORIES PER SERVING: 370

1 large red onion, finely chopped

low-calorie cooking spray

2 garlic cloves, crushed

800g (1lb 12oz) sweet potato, peeled and chopped into smallish cubes

1 teaspoon smoked paprika, plus extra to serve

1 teaspoon ground cumin

1 teaspoon dried oregano

400ml (14fl oz) vegetable stock

400g (14oz) can chopped tomatoes

1 tablespoon tomato purée

2 × 400g (14oz) cans black beans, drained and rinsed

40g (1½oz) pickled jalapeños, finely chopped

salt and pepper

lime wedges, to serve

fat-free yogurt, to serve

1. In a large sauté pan with a lid, fry the onion gently in low-calorie cooking spray for 5 minutes, then add the garlic, sweet potato, smoked paprika, cumin and oregano and stir-fry for a couple of minutes.
2. Pour in the stock, then add the tomatoes, tomato purée, black beans and jalapeños. Season with salt and pepper.
3. Simmer gently for 30 minutes, stirring occasionally, then place a lid on the pan and cook over a low heat for another 15 minutes.
4. Check the sweet potato chunks are cooked through, then serve with lime wedges, and fat-free yogurt sprinkled with smoked paprika.

NOTE If you prefer, you can replace the sweet potato with butternut squash, and stir in some spinach or kale at the end of cooking. To make this extra tasty, top with grated cheese at the end of cooking and grill under a hot grill until browned and bubbling (make sure your pan is ovenproof first).

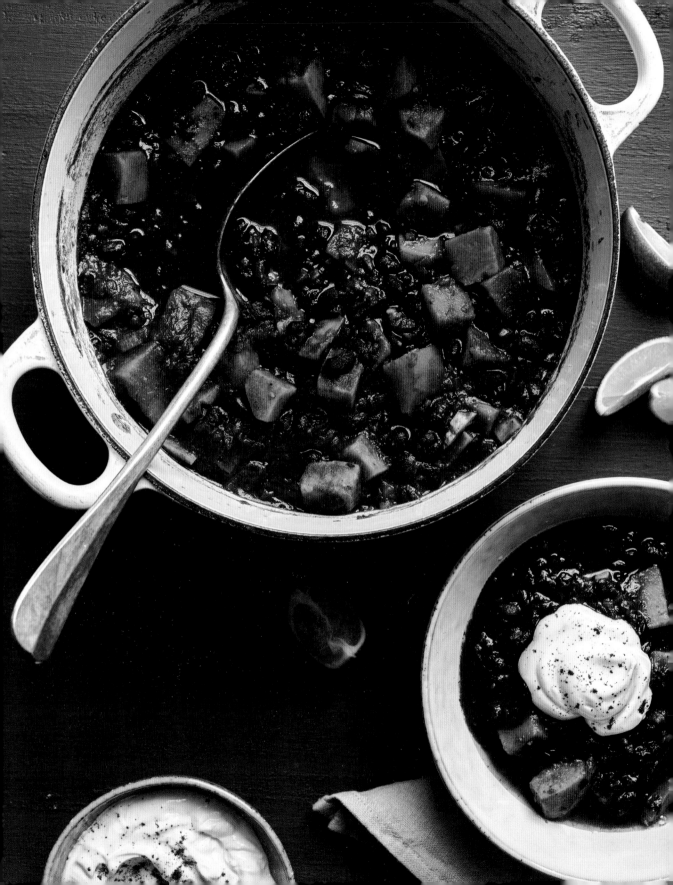

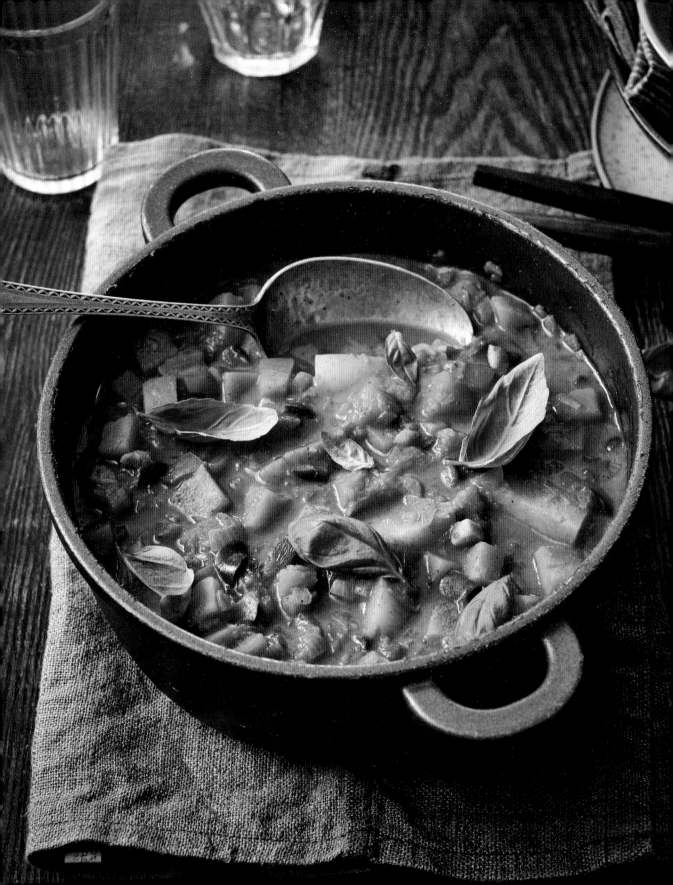

CREAMY COCONUT, BUTTERNUT SQUASH & POTATO THAI RED CURRY

One of the tastiest soups I have ever eaten was a creamy, spiced tomato and coconut milk soup at a Thai restaurant in London. Here I've recreated those flavours in a Thai curry, using light coconut milk, which has less than half the fat of regular, but still gives a lovely creaminess.

CALORIES PER SERVING: 261

2 onions, finely chopped

low-calorie cooking spray

2 garlic cloves, crushed

1 red pepper, deseeded and finely chopped

2 tablespoons Thai red curry paste

400g (14oz) can light coconut milk

3 tablespoons tomato purée

1 tablespoon dark soy sauce

juice of 1 lime

½ teaspoon salt

500g (1lb 2oz) butternut squash, peeled, deseeded and chopped into rough 1cm (½ inch) cubes

500g (1lb 2oz) new potatoes, quartered (no need to peel)

handful of basil leaves, to serve

1. In a sauté pan or deep frying pan, fry the onions gently in low-calorie cooking spray for 10 minutes, until softened and a light golden colour.

2. Add the garlic and red pepper and stir-fry over a slightly higher heat for 1 minute.

3. Stir in the curry paste until the vegetables are coated, then pour in the coconut milk. Fill up the can with water and add that too.

4. Now squeeze in the tomato purée and add the soy sauce, lime juice, salt, squash and potatoes. Bring up to a rapid simmer, mixing everything together.

5. Reduce the heat to a gentle simmer. Cook for 40 minutes, stirring occasionally.

6. When it's ready, the sauce will be thick and creamy and the vegetables cooked through.

7. Scatter the basil leaves over and serve.

NOTE You can freeze raw butternut squash, so if you have some left over, simply peel, chop and put it into a freezer bag or sealed container to freeze. This can then be used for a quick soup or curry when you need it. Serve this curry on its own or with cauliflower 'rice' (see page 148).

COD PUTTANESCA WITH BROKEN SPAGHETTI

The combination of flavours in puttanesca sauce is mouth-wateringly good. Salty anchovies with chilli and garlic make the perfect base for a savoury tomato sauce and I love the little pops of flavour that come from the olives and capers here.

CALORIES PER SERVING: 412

50g (1¾oz) can anchovies in olive oil, fully drained

3 garlic cloves, crushed

1 red chilli, deseeded and finely chopped

2 teaspoons dried oregano

1 teaspoon finely chopped rosemary leaves, plus extra to serve

6 sage leaves, finely chopped, plus extra to serve

2 × 400g (14oz) cans chopped tomatoes

1 tablespoon tomato purée

350ml (12fl oz) water

250g (9oz) dried spaghetti, strands broken into quarters

16 pitted black olives (about 40g / 1½oz), sliced

2 tablespoons capers

4 frozen cod fillets

salt and pepper

1. Dab the anchovies with kitchen paper to remove excess oil, roughly chop them, then fry them in a large deep pan for 2 minutes with the garlic and chilli, breaking up the anchovies with a wooden spoon. You won't need cooking spray, as there is enough residual oil in the anchovies.

2. Add the oregano, rosemary and sage and stir-fry for about 30 seconds, then add the tomatoes, tomato purée and measured water. Bring up to a rapid simmer, then tip in the broken spaghetti. Give this a good stir around to ensure that the strands are separated, then add the olives and capers.

3. Lay the frozen fish fillets on top of the stew, season with salt and pepper, pop a lid on and leave to simmer for 15 minutes.

4. Remove the lid and use a fork to shuffle the pasta about (being careful not to break up the fish), just to ensure it isn't clumping.

5. Simmer for 5 more minutes, then check the spaghetti is cooked through. It should be al dente, but not hard.

6. Serve immediately, scattered with more rosemary and sage.

NOTE If you are using fresh, not frozen, fish, place the fillets on top of the stew when there is about 6 minutes of cooking time remaining.

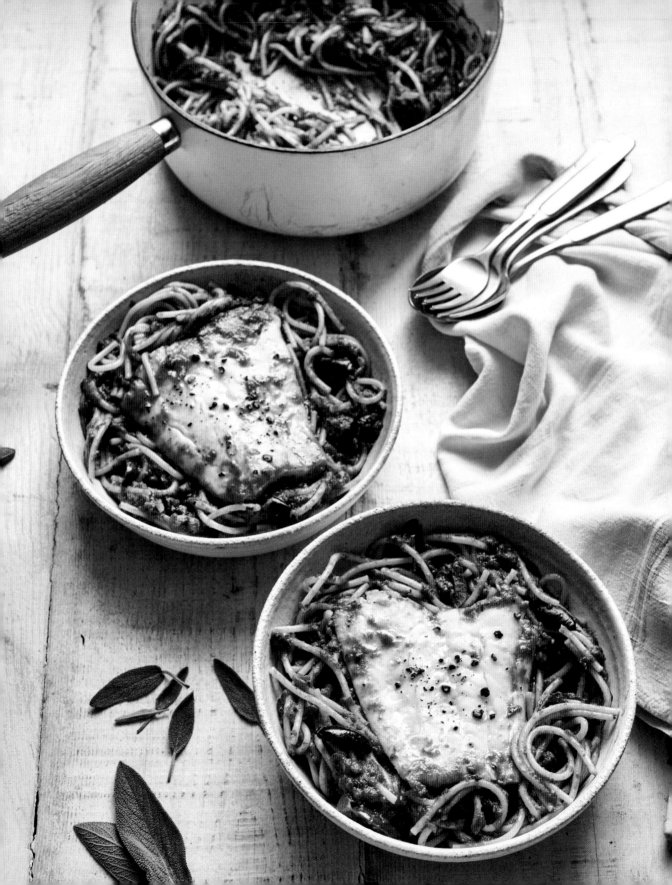

EASY SPANISH CHICKEN & CHORIZO STEW

A rustic one-pot with vibrant sweet and smoky flavours, packed with healthy vegetables and with the filling power of creamy butter beans. One of the things I love about chorizo is that you can get so much flavour from just a small amount. Serve this on its own, with some crusty bread or with rice or couscous.

CALORIES PER SERVING: 413

50g (1¾oz) chorizo, very finely chopped

3 chicken breasts, chopped

2 red onions, finely chopped

4 garlic cloves, crushed

2 celery sticks, finely chopped

2 carrots, peeled and finely chopped

1 yellow pepper, deseeded and chopped

1 red pepper, deseeded and chopped

800ml (1 pint 8fl oz) chicken stock

2 × 400g (14oz) cans butter beans, drained and rinsed

1 tablespoon smoked paprika

1 tablespoon dried thyme

2 tablespoons tomato purée

juice of ½ lemon

large handful of parsley leaves, finely chopped

1. In a large casserole dish with a lid, fry the chorizo for 2 minutes until sizzling and starting to colour.
2. Add the chicken and stir-fry for 5 minutes until no pink is showing.
3. Add the onions, garlic, celery, carrots and peppers and place the lid on. Leave to cook gently on a low heat for 10 minutes, stirring occasionally.
4. Pour in the stock, add the butter beans, smoked paprika, thyme and tomato purée, stir everything together, then leave to simmer gently, uncovered, for 30 minutes, giving it the occasional stir.
5. When you're ready to serve, add the lemon juice and most of the chopped parsley, give it a good stir, then sprinkle the rest of the parsley over the top.

NOTE You can replace the chicken with pork, or sausage if you prefer, and – to add a little more Spanish flavour – scatter in a handful of olives.

YELLOW SPLIT PEA DHAL

Simply spiced sweet and mellow split peas create a warming bowl of comfort food. Serve on their own, with rice or with freshly cooked Quick & Easy Wholemeal 3-ingredient Flatbreads (see page 188).

CALORIES PER SERVING: 252

low-calorie cooking spray
1 onion, finely chopped
1 red chilli, finely chopped
1½ teaspoons cumin seeds
250g (9oz) dried yellow split peas
700ml (1¼ pints) vegetable stock
1 teaspoon ground turmeric
½ teaspoon chilli powder
½ teaspoon salt

1. Spray a large casserole with low-calorie cooking spray, add the onion and fry gently for 10 minutes. Add the red chilli and cumin seeds and stir-fry for 1 minute.
2. Give the split peas a good rinse in a sieve, then add them to the casserole. Cover with the stock, stir in the turmeric, chilli powder and salt and bring up to a rapid simmer.
3. Cover the pot, reduce the temperature to low so the peas are just gently simmering, and simmer for 45 minutes, giving them a stir halfway through.
4. Taste to check that the peas are cooked through with no bite, cooking for a little longer if needed, and add a dash of boiling water if the dhal is starting to get too dry. Serve immediately.

NOTE This is also tasty with cauliflower – just add some florets 10 minutes before the dhal has finished cooking, placing the lid back on so the cauliflower steams in with the dhal.

SLOW-COOKER HONEY GARLIC CHICKEN

This is an all-round favourite on the blog, and for good reason! It only takes a few minutes and minimal effort to pull together, but it tastes great. Cooking it all together in one pot means there is no need for oil and there is just enough honey to add a lovely sweetness without making it overly sugary. After cooking, the chicken is tender enough to pull apart into the honey and garlic sauce. It's a really versatile dish and can be served with stir-fried vegetables, salad, brown rice, noodles or in a wrap.

CALORIES PER SERVING: 230

2 tablespoons honey

2 tablespoons tomato purée

2 tablespoons dark soy sauce

1 tablespoon rice vinegar

2 tablespoons water

6 spring onions, trimmed and finely sliced

6 garlic cloves, crushed

4 chicken breasts

1 tablespoon sesame seeds

handful of coriander leaves, to serve

1. In a small bowl, mix together the honey, tomato purée, soy sauce, rice vinegar and measured water. Stir in the spring onions and crushed garlic.

2. Pop the chicken breasts into the slow cooker bowl and cover with the sauce. Put the lid on.

3. Cook on high for 2–3 hours, or on low for 4–5 hours, stirring halfway through.

4. The chicken should now pull apart easily and you can shred it into the sauce using 2 forks.

5. To serve, dry-fry the sesame seeds for a couple of minutes to give them a little bit of colour and a toasty flavour, then sprinkle over the top of the chicken. Scatter with the coriander leaves.

NOTE To cook this in the oven instead, place all the ingredients in a casserole dish with a lid and bake in an oven preheated to 210°C/190°C fan (410°F), Gas Mark 6½, for 45 minutes.

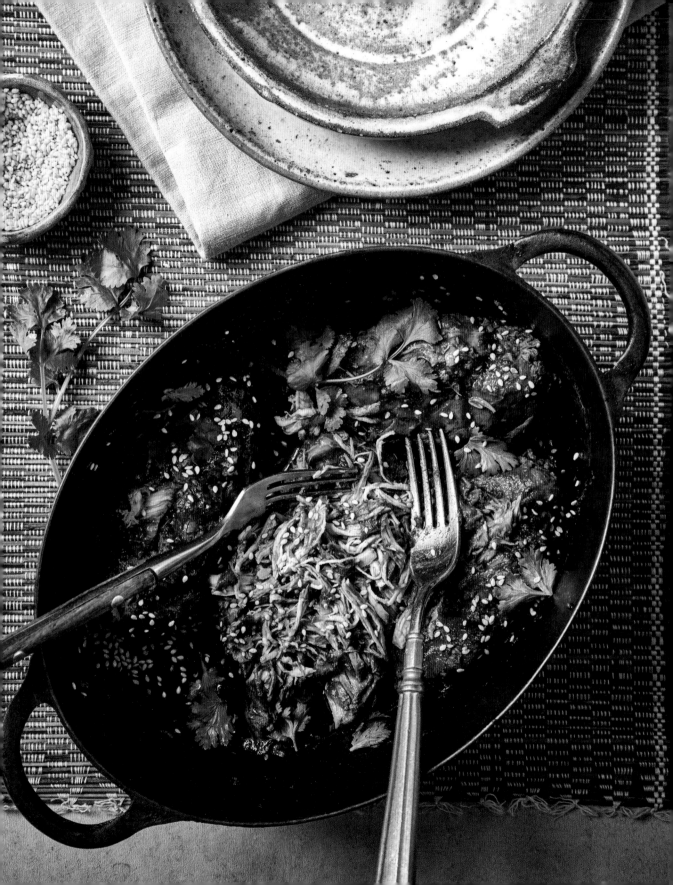

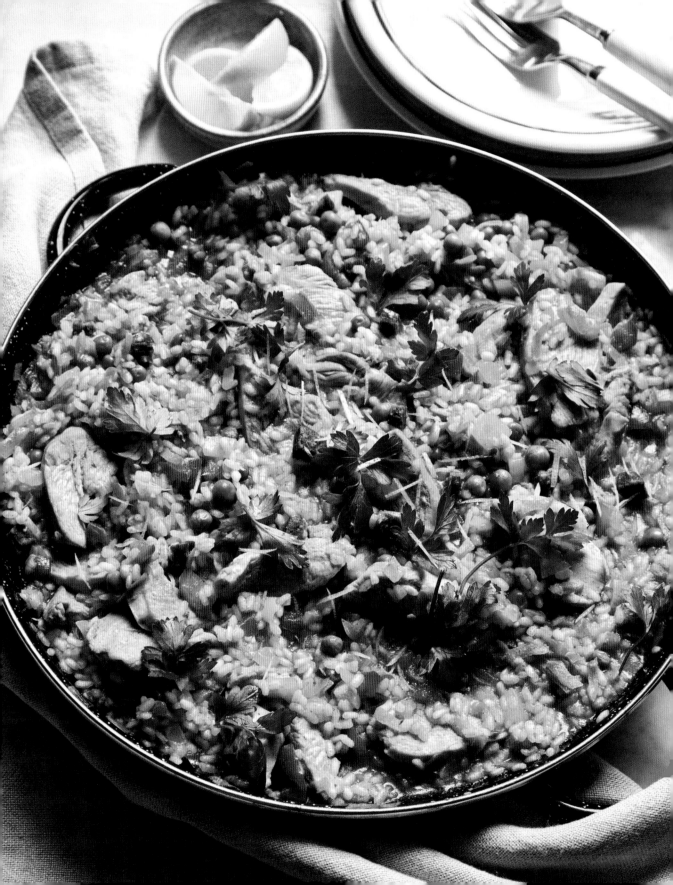

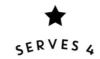

ZESTY CHICKEN & CHORIZO PAELLA

Bursting with the flavours of zingy lemon and smoky chorizo, this simple paella is always a crowd-pleaser. If you can't get hold of paella rice, simply substitute with Arborio rice or even long-grain rice. Serve some green vegetables, such as green beans or broccoli, alongside.

CALORIES PER SERVING: 490

1 teaspoon rapeseed oil

35g (1¼oz) chorizo, finely chopped

3 chicken breasts, chopped into chunks

1 onion, finely chopped

2 garlic cloves, finely chopped

15g (½oz) parsley, leaves separated, stalks chopped

1 carrot, peeled and grated

1 red pepper, deseeded and chopped

1 teaspoon smoked paprika

½ teaspoon cayenne pepper

½ teaspoon ground turmeric

1 chicken stock cube

300g (10½oz) paella rice (or see recipe introduction)

750ml (1⅓ pints) boiling water

100g (3½oz) frozen peas

1 lemon

salt and pepper

1. Heat the oil in a large wok or similar pan. Add the chorizo, chicken, onion, garlic, parsley stalks and grated carrot and stir-fry for 5 minutes.
2. Add in the red pepper, paprika, cayenne pepper and turmeric and stir-fry for another 3 minutes.
3. Crumble in the chicken stock cube, then stir in the rice until thoroughly combined with all of the other ingredients. Pour in the measured boiling water and leave to simmer for about 5 minutes.
4. Stir, then simmer for another 10 minutes, stirring regularly to prevent sticking.
5. Add the peas, season with salt and pepper and stir-fry for a final 5 minutes.
6. Check that the rice is cooked and not chalky. Grate the lemon zest directly over the top of the dish and scatter with the parsley leaves. Chop the lemon into wedges and serve on the side.

NOTE If you fancy adding some prawns, simply fry them separately and stir them in when the paella is cooked.

COWGIRLS' STEW

This is a great, family-friendly dish, one of the easiest and quickest-to-prepare recipes in the book. It's full of smoky, barbecue-scented meat that makes you feel as though you're sitting around a campfire! Serve in a bowl on its own, with jacket potatoes and corn on the cob, or over brown rice.

CALORIES PER SERVING: 369

1 red onion, finely chopped

2 garlic cloves, crushed

2 celery sticks, finely chopped

1 red pepper, deseeded and chopped

1 green pepper, deseeded and chopped

400g (14oz) can chopped tomatoes

400g (14oz) can haricot beans, drained and rinsed

400g (14oz) can cannellini beans, drained and rinsed

1 beef stock cube

150ml (¼ pint) boiling water

6 tablespoons tomato purée

6 tablespoons shop-bought barbecue sauce

1 tablespoon smoked paprika

1 teaspoon salt

¼ teaspoon pepper

1 pork fillet, about 450g (1lb)

1. Put all of the ingredients, apart from the pork, into the slow cooker bowl and stir together.
2. Place the pork fillet in the pot, put on the lid and cook on high for 6–8 hours, or low for 10–12 hours.
3. Once cooked, use 2 forks to break up and pull apart the pork and mix it through the stew. Serve immediately.

NOTE Fancy a bit of spice? Stir in some finely chopped pickled jalapeños once the stew is cooked. If you would like to cook this in the oven, place all the ingredients in a casserole dish with a lid and cook for 1½ hours in an oven preheated to 200°C/180°C fan (400°F), Gas Mark 6.

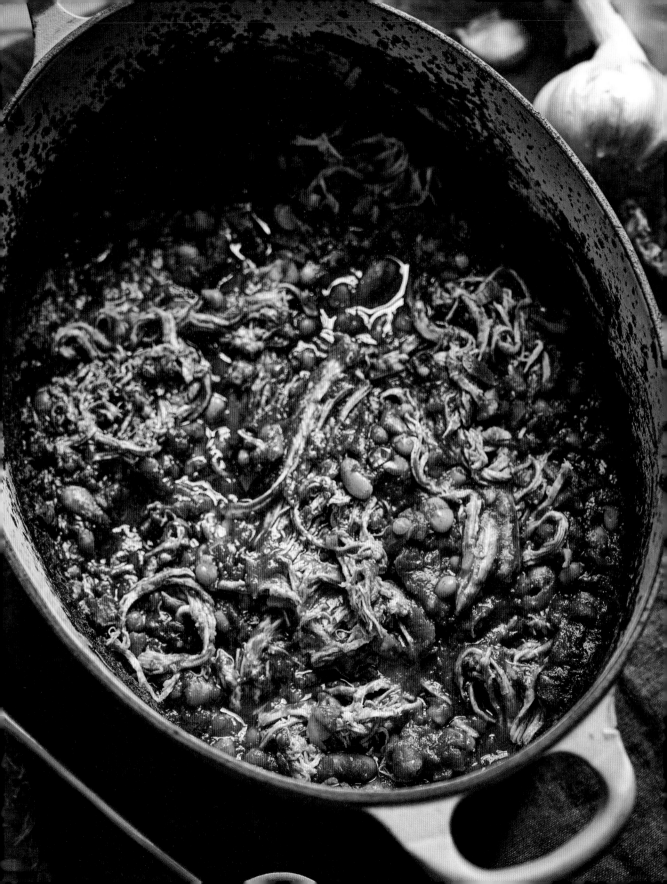

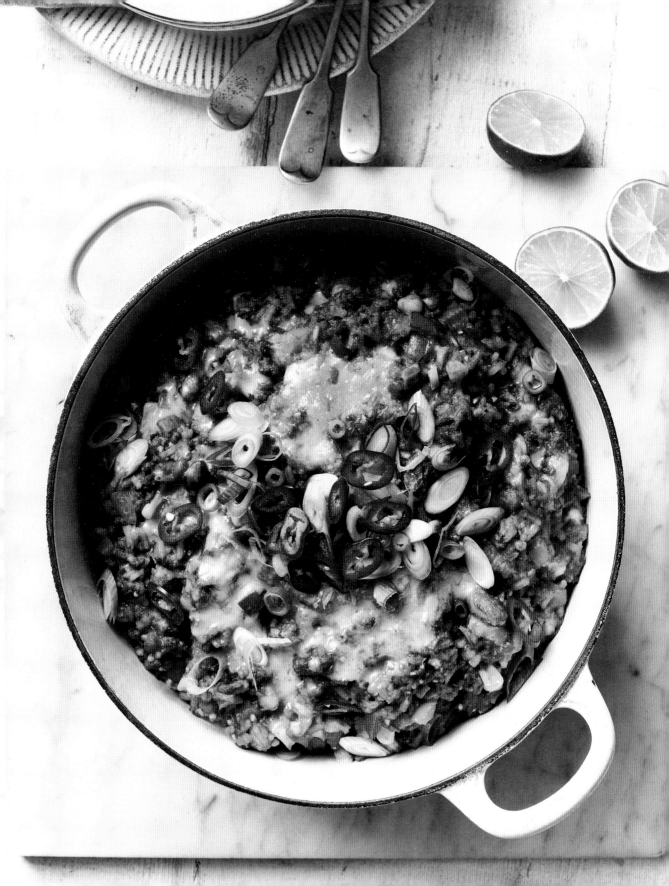

FIESTA BEEF

I often make a big batch of this hearty Mexican-inspired dish and save some in the freezer to be easily reheated for weekday lunches.

CALORIES PER SERVING: 432

low-calorie cooking spray

1 onion, finely chopped

2 garlic cloves, crushed

500g (1lb 2oz) lean minced beef (less than 5 per cent fat)

1 red pepper, chopped

1 yellow pepper, chopped

2 tablespoons Taco spice mix (see page 212)

160g (5¾oz) long-grain white rice

500ml (18fl oz) beef stock

400g (14oz) can chopped tomatoes

400g (14oz) can pinto beans, drained and rinsed

juice of 1 lime, plus extra lime wedges, to serve

100g (3½oz) frozen sweetcorn

125ml (4fl oz) semi-skimmed milk

100g (3½oz) Cheddar cheese, grated

TO SERVE
sliced spring onions
chopped red chilli

1. Spray a large casserole dish with low-calorie cooking spray and fry the onion, garlic and beef gently for 8 minutes, breaking up the minced meat with a wooden spoon.
2. Stir in the spice mix and cook for about 1 minute, then stir in the peppers.
3. Add the rice, stir it through, then pour in the stock.
4. Tip in the tomatoes, beans, lime juice and sweetcorn and simmer for 20 minutes, giving it a stir every now and again.
5. Preheat the grill on its highest setting.
6. Check that the rice is cooked, then stir in the milk with three-quarters of the grated cheese.
7. Sprinkle the remaining cheese over the top, then place under the hot grill for 4 minutes, until the cheese is golden and bubbling.
8. Sprinkle with the spring onions and red chilli, and serve with lime wedges.

NOTE This dish can easily be made vegetarian by swapping the beef for black beans, and the beef stock for vegetable stock. You can also serve this alongside crunchy shredded lettuce with a fresh lime dressing.

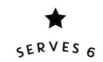

SERVES 6

CHILLI MAC'N'CHEESE

This all-in-one dish is the perfect comfort food and is packed full of Mexican flavours. It's great for feeding a crowd and reheats well too.

CALORIES PER SERVING: 519

low-calorie cooking spray
1 onion, finely chopped
2 garlic cloves, crushed
2 red peppers, chopped
500g (1lb 2oz) lean minced beef (less than 5 per cent fat)
400g (14oz) can chopped tomatoes
1 tablespoon tomato purée
400g can red kidney beans, drained and rinsed
1 tablespoon Worcestershire sauce
800ml (1¾ pints) beef stock
300g (10½oz) dried macaroni
175g (6oz) Cheddar cheese, finely grated

FOR THE SPICE MIX
1 teaspoon chilli powder
2 teaspoons paprika
1 teaspoon ground cumin
1 teaspoon onion granules
1 teaspoon dried oregano
½ teaspoon pepper
1 teaspoon salt

1. Get your spice mix ready by mixing all the spices together in a small bowl.
2. Spray a large, ovenproof saucepan or casserole dish with low-calorie cooking spray and fry the onion and garlic gently for 3 minutes.
3. Add the red peppers to the pan and fry for 1 more minute.
4. Add the minced meat and cook until brown, stirring and breaking it up with a spoon, then spoon in the spice mix and stir it through the meat thoroughly.
5. Add the tomatoes, tomato purée, kidney beans and Worcestershire sauce. Stir again.
6. Pour in the beef stock and the macaroni and stir well. Put the lid on and simmer gently for 15 minutes, until the macaroni is cooked. For the last few minutes, remove the lid and bubble gently, giving it a good stir. Preheat the grill on its highest setting.
7. Remove from the heat and stir in half the cheese.
8. Sprinkle the rest of the cheese on top and place under the hot grill for about 5 minutes, until the cheese is bubbling, melted and browned on top.

NOTE Not a fan of kidney beans? Replace them with black beans, pinto beans or haricot beans. If you fancy some more oozy, stringy cheese, stir some mozzarella through the pot before scattering the Cheddar on top and grilling.

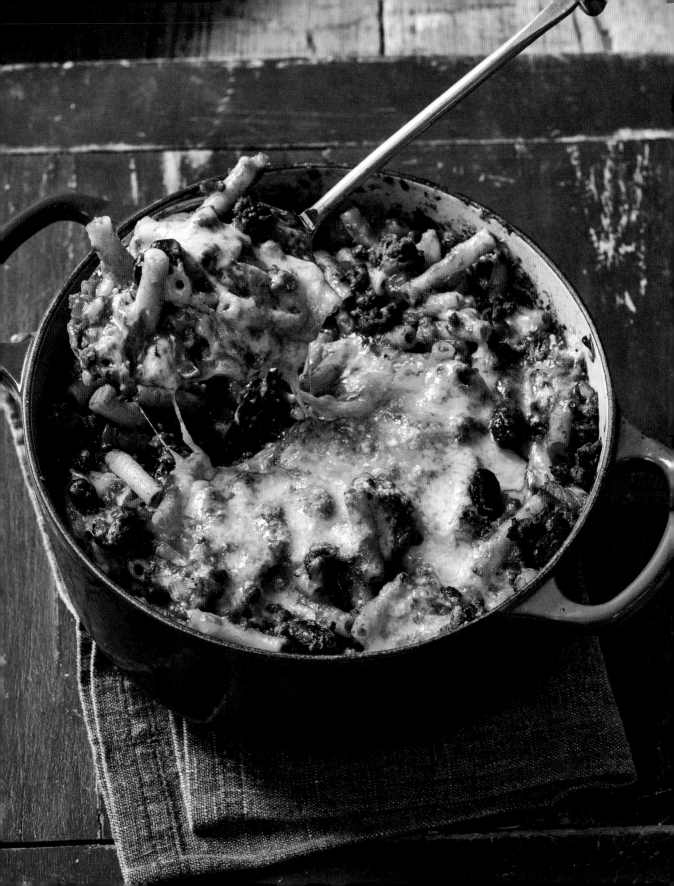

SAVOURY TRAYBAKES

• • • • • • • • • • • • •

Savoury traybakes are a great way to make simple, fuss-free meals that don't require lots of hands-on cooking. Roasting really draws out the flavours of a lot of ingredients and adds another dimension, making many meals even more delicious. I started making my Flaming Fajita Traybake a few years ago, as I found that you still got the characteristic flavours of fried onions and peppers without standing over a hot stove, which also gives you time to create some side dishes to serve alongside.

Making a traybaked soup is a great use of this technique – you can just pop all the ingredients in and leave them to cook – and vegetables such as carrot and ginger are really enhanced in this way.

Because some traybakes can be prepared in advance, they work particularly well when cooking for friends. The Classic Sloppy Joe, traybake style, makes a fun centrepiece if you're feeding a group.

The recipes in this chapter explore different textures, flavours and cuisines from around the world, with some lighter options for lunches and others more suited to a main evening meal. Most of them are family-friendly; my children especially love the Garlicky Meatball Pasta Bake and the Piggy-in-the-middle.

• • • • • • • • • • • • •

GREEK-STYLE ORZO
WITH BAKED FETA

The quick cooking time and rice-like size and shape of orzo mean it's perfectly suited to traybakes. The light and fresh flavours in this pasta bake, with lots of healthy vegetables included, is complemented by salty baked feta and the satisfying crunch of sunflower seeds. Serve with a simple green salad.

CALORIES PER SERVING: 416

---

1 onion, finely chopped

2 garlic cloves, finely chopped

1 red pepper, deseeded and chopped

150g (5½oz) cherry tomatoes, halved

finely grated zest and juice of 1 unwaxed lemon

1 tablespoon dried oregano

low-calorie cooking spray

300g (10½oz) dried orzo pasta

small handful of mint leaves, finely chopped

50g (1¾oz) baby spinach

800ml (1¾ pints) vegetable stock

90g (3¼oz) feta cheese, cut into small chunks

2 tablespoons sunflower seeds

salt and pepper

1. Preheat the oven to 220°C/200°C fan (425°F), Gas Mark 7.

2. Place the onion, garlic, pepper and tomatoes into a deep baking tray or casserole dish and stir in the lemon zest and juice and oregano. Spray with low-calorie cooking spray and bake in the oven for 15 minutes.

3. Remove from the oven and stir through the orzo, add in the mint and spinach, season with salt and pepper, then pour in the stock. Stir again and bake in the oven for 15 minutes.

4. Remove from the oven, give the orzo a stir, cover the top evenly with the feta, then sprinkle over the sunflower seeds.

5. Bake for 10 minutes. The orzo should be cooked through with no bite, the feta melted and starting to brown a little, and the sunflower seeds golden brown.

NOTE This recipe also works very nicely with roasted peppers from a jar, rather than fresh peppers. Simply slice a few up and stir them in after the orzo has cooked, just before topping with the feta and sunflower seeds.

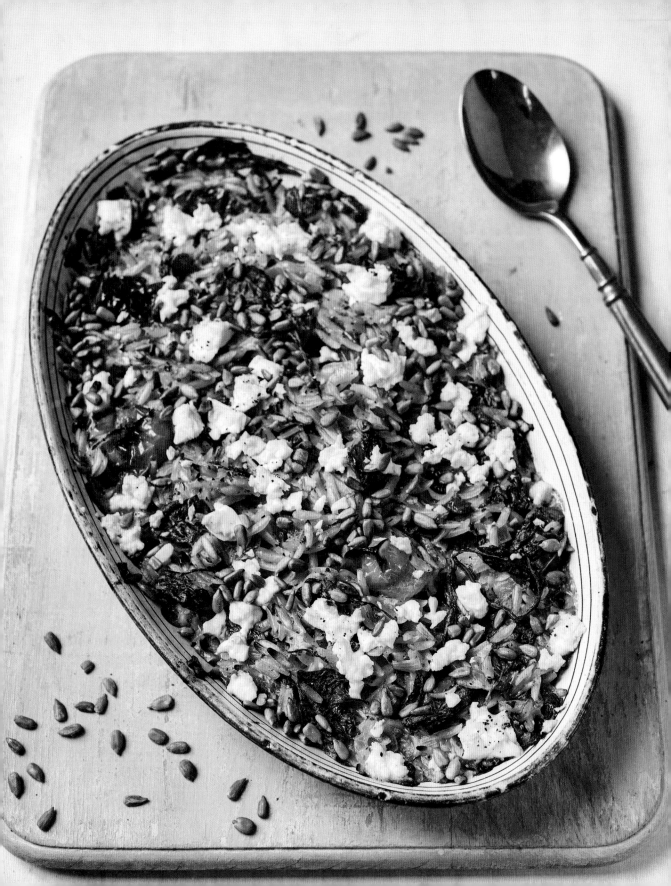

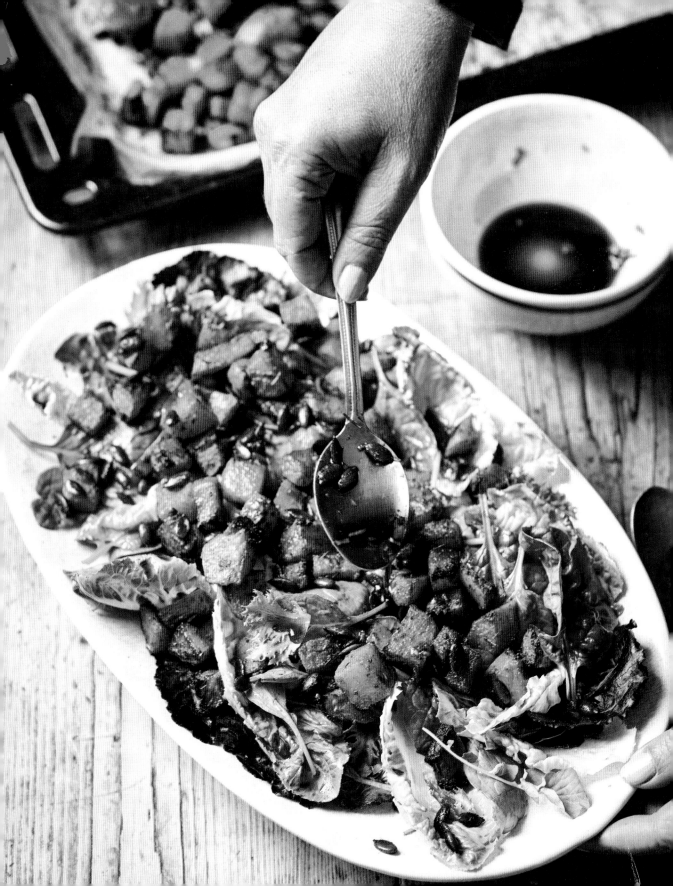

WARM SPICED SQUASH & PUMPKIN SEED SALAD

Butternut squash is a real hero ingredient. When bought whole it has a long shelf life, so it's always worth keeping one in, 'just in case'. It's rich in fibre and vitamins, and so versatile. Roasted in cubes for this dish, it is tender, sweet and has great filling power. This is a satisfying salad for any season.

CALORIES PER SERVING: 150

low-calorie cooking spray
750g (1lb 10oz) butternut squash, peeled, deseeded and cut into small cubes (about 2cm / ¾ inch)
1 teaspoon paprika
½ teaspoon cayenne pepper
½ teaspoon ground cumin
½ teaspoon dried thyme
4 tablespoons pumpkin seeds
175g (6oz) mixed salad leaves
salt and pepper

FOR THE DRESSING
1 tablespoon balsamic vinegar
1 tablespoon soy sauce
1 teaspoon honey
1 garlic clove, crushed

1. Preheat the oven to 220°C/200°C fan (425°F), Gas Mark 7.
2. Line a large baking tray with baking parchment, spray it with low-calorie cooking spray and spread the butternut squash cubes out. Sprinkle over the paprika, cayenne pepper, cumin and thyme, season with salt and pepper, and mix well so the squash is coated with the spices.
3. Scatter over the pumpkin seeds, then spray generously with cooking spray.
4. Roast for 30 minutes, until the squash is tender and has golden brown edges.
5. Remove from the oven and allow to cool slightly while you make the dressing.
6. In a small bowl, mix up the balsamic vinegar, soy sauce, honey and garlic.
7. Empty the salad leaves into a large serving bowl, add the contents of the baking tray and toss everything together.
8. Drizzle the dressing over and serve immediately.

NOTE Sweet potato can be used as well as (or instead of) butternut squash in this salad. Around Halloween, when pumpkins are plentiful and cheap, use those instead.

EMPTY-THE-FRIDGE FRITTATA

This is a great way to avoid food waste and use up the odd tomato or mushroom lurking in the refrigerator, or any leftover veg from a previous meal. A fluffy, light baked frittata is a great lunch option if you are feeding lots of people, as the recipe can easily be scaled up and you can make it in advance. Serve with a fresh salad.

CALORIES PER SERVING: 250

1 onion, finely chopped

1 red pepper, deseeded and finely chopped

100g (3½oz) cherry tomatoes, halved

low-calorie cooking spray

1 large handful (about 40g / 1½oz) baby spinach

8 eggs

125ml (4fl oz) semi-skimmed milk

40g (1½oz) Cheddar cheese, grated

salt and pepper

1. Preheat the oven to 200°C/180°C fan (400°F), Gas Mark 6.
2. Fry the onion, pepper and tomatoes together in low-calorie cooking spray for 7 minutes, until softened and the onions are starting to go golden brown. Remove from the heat and stir in the spinach until it wilts. Season with salt and pepper.
3. Line a 30 x 20cm (12 x 8 inch) roasting tin with baking parchment and spread the cooked vegetables on top.
4. Whisk together the eggs and milk in a bowl, then stir in half the cheese.
5. Pour the egg mixture over the vegetables, then sprinkle with the remaining cheese.
6. Bake for 20 minutes, until light golden brown on top and set in the middle. The frittata should be light and fluffy.

NOTE You can tailor this to use up whatever you have. For vegetables that require a little more cooking – such as mushrooms, leeks, courgettes and broccoli – fry them alongside any onions or shallots for a few minutes. Vegetables such as green beans, peas, asparagus or broad beans (plus any leftover herbs that need using) can just be added when you pour the egg mixture into the tray. Odds and ends of different cheeses can be used too – why not try feta, goats' cheese, mozzarella or Parmesan?

FRAGRANT TRAYBAKED CARROT & GINGER SOUP

Comforting and nourishing, the ginger in this recipe perfectly complements the sweetness of the carrot. I love to make soup in this way – it saves any pre-frying and means you can just throw in all the ingredients and leave it to cook.

CALORIES PER SERVING: 84

1 onion, quartered

1 tablespoon peeled and finely chopped fresh root ginger

2 garlic cloves, peeled

500g (1lb 2oz) carrots, peeled and roughly chopped

finely grated zest and juice of 1 medium-sized orange

low-calorie cooking spray

1 litre (1¾ pints) vegetable stock

½ teaspoon salt

pepper

handful of parsley leaves, finely chopped, to serve

1. Preheat the oven to 220°C/200°C (425°F), Gas Mark 7.
2. Throw the onion quarters into a deep baking tray, add the ginger, garlic, carrots, orange zest and juice, give everything a good mix, then spray with low-calorie cooking spray.
3. Put on the middle shelf of the oven and roast for 30 minutes.
4. Reduce the oven temperature to 200°C/180°C fan (400°F), Gas Mark 6, remove the baking tray from the oven, give the vegetables a good stir, then pour in the stock.
5. Return the tray to the oven for another 30 minutes.
6. Using a hand blender or a food processor, blend the soup until smooth, adding the salt.
7. Serve with a little bit of black pepper ground on top, and sprinkled with parsley.

NOTE Use a teaspoon to scrape the skin from the ginger easily.

ITALIAN CHICKEN CACCIATORE

I first tried chicken cacciatore in an American-Italian restaurant and I was instantly a huge fan of the rich, vegetable-packed herby tomato sauce, so I turned it into a traybake to simplify the process.

CALORIES PER SERVING: 385

2 red onions, finely chopped

4 garlic cloves, crushed

1 red pepper, deseeded and chopped

1 yellow pepper, deseeded and chopped

2 celery sticks, finely chopped

125g (4½oz) chestnut mushrooms, quartered

200g (7oz) cherry tomatoes, halved

2 tablespoons balsamic vinegar

2 tablespoons Italian mixed herbs

low-calorie cooking spray

400g (14oz) can chopped tomatoes

250g (9oz) tomato passata

8 chicken thigh fillets, fat trimmed away

1 teaspoon salt

pepper

finely chopped fresh herbs, to serve

1. Preheat the oven to 220°C/200°C fan (425°F), Gas Mark 7.
2. Place the onions, garlic, peppers, celery, mushrooms, cherry tomatoes, balsamic vinegar and Italian mixed herbs into a deep baking tray or large ovenproof dish, spray with low-calorie cooking spray and roast for 15 minutes.
3. Remove from the oven, give the vegetables a stir, then add the chopped tomatoes, passata and chicken, and season with the salt and some pepper. Give everything a good stir and return to the oven for 20 minutes.
4. Serve scattered with fresh herbs. I like to use parsley, basil and oregano, but you can use whatever you have in.

NOTE This is a great dish for scaling up to feed lots of people if you have a nice big baking tray! You can just prepare the vegetables in advance, put them in the tray and cover with foil until you are ready to bake it. There's very little work once all the preparation has been done. You can serve it with pasta if you like but, for a lighter accompaniment, try it with Cannellini Bean Mash (see page 147) or a rocket salad.

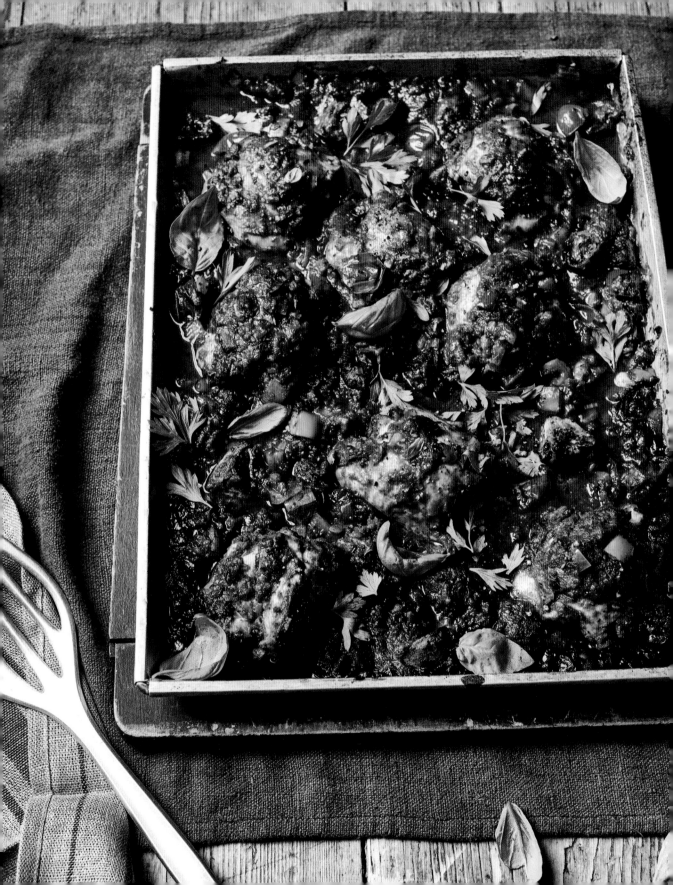

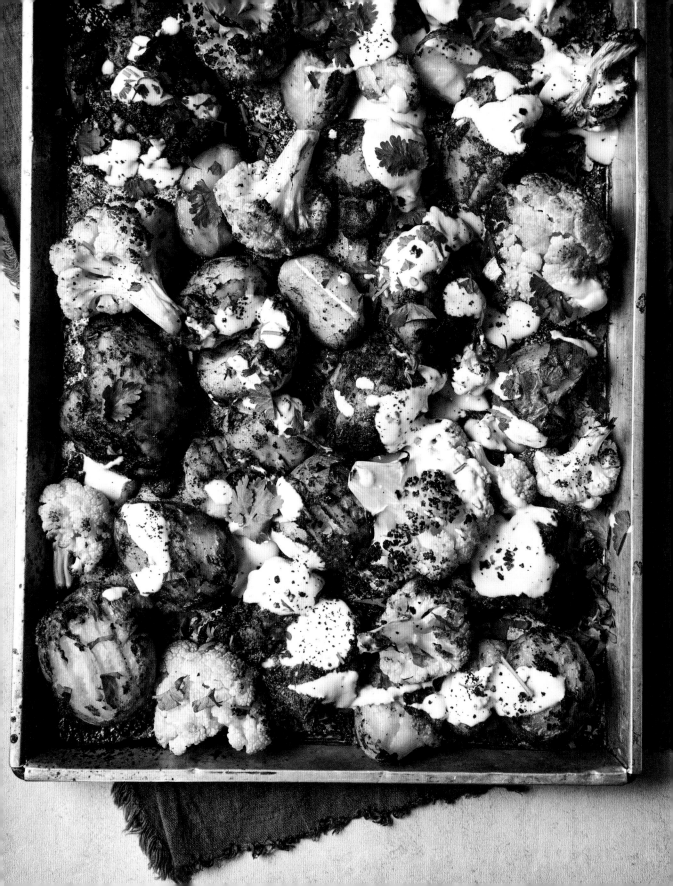

SUMAC CHICKEN, POTATO & CAULIFLOWER

This is a versatile traybake that works for every season – a warming dish for winter, but with Mediterranean flavours that also work well in the summer. Serve with green beans, asparagus, Ribboned Courgette & Zesty Lemon Salad (see page 134) or a simple salad.

CALORIES PER SERVING: 523

700g (1lb 9oz) new potatoes (no need to peel)
2 teaspoons sumac
1 teaspoon chilli flakes
1 teaspoon dried thyme
1 teaspoon ground cumin
½ teaspoon ground cinnamon
1 tablespoon tomato purée
2 tablespoons red wine vinegar
3 tablespoons fat-free Greek yogurt
8 skinless chicken thigh fillets
low-calorie cooking spray
1 cauliflower, leaves and stem removed, florets separated
handful of coriander leaves, roughly chopped
salt and pepper

1. Preheat the oven to 220°C/200°C fan (425°F), Gas Mark 7.
2. Put the potatoes in a large saucepan of boiling water and simmer for 15 minutes.
3. Meanwhile, in a large bowl, mix up the sumac, chilli, thyme, cumin, cinnamon, tomato purée, red wine vinegar and 1 tablespoon of the Greek yogurt, then add the chicken and turn to fully coat in the marinade.
4. Drain the potatoes, spray a deep baking tray or ovenproof casserole dish with low-calorie cooking spray, add the potatoes and use a potato masher to crush them. The aim is not to mash them completely, but to partly flatten and burst them. If a few edges get mashed, then don't worry, these just add tasty little crispy bits.
5. Place the marinated chicken in the tray in the gaps between the potatoes. Spray generously with cooking spray.
6. Place on the top shelf of the oven for 20 minutes.
7. Remove the tray from the oven, stir the potatoes and chicken to mix them up and turn them over, then add the cauliflower. Spray again with cooking spray, season with salt and pepper, and roast on the top shelf of the oven for 10 minutes.
8. Remove from the oven, drizzle over the remaining Greek yogurt and sprinkle with chopped coriander. Serve immediately.

NOTE Try adding some extra vegetables to cook for the final 10 minutes, such as green beans, broccoli or courgettes.

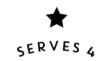

FLAMING FAJITA TRAYBAKE

Satisfying, spicy chicken fajita mix is so easy to make with the traybake method. Simply chuck in all the ingredients and then it's hands off until they are ready! Serve in wraps or with rice and black beans. This is also gorgeous with homemade Zucchimole (see page 208).

CALORIES PER SERVING: 188

low-calorie cooking spray
2 onions, halved, then sliced
3 peppers (I use red, orange and yellow), deseeded and cut into strips
3 chicken breasts, sliced into strips
2 tablespoons Fajita spice mix (see page 212)

TO SERVE
handful of coriander leaves
lime wedges

1. Preheat the oven to 200°C/180°C fan (400°F), Gas Mark 6.
2. Spray the base of a deep, nonstick baking tray with low-calorie cooking spray and spread the onions, peppers and chicken over in an even layer.
3. Sprinkle the spice mix over the top and give everything a shuffle around to coat in the spices.
4. Spray with cooking spray.
5. Put the baking tray into the oven and bake for 35 minutes until the chicken is cooked through and the peppers and onions are cooked and very slightly charred.
6. Serve with coriander and lime wedges.

NOTE Make this dish vegetarian by replacing the chicken with butternut squash or sweet potato. You can bulk it out by stirring in some drained canned beans, such as black beans or pinto beans, 5 minutes before the end of the cooking time.

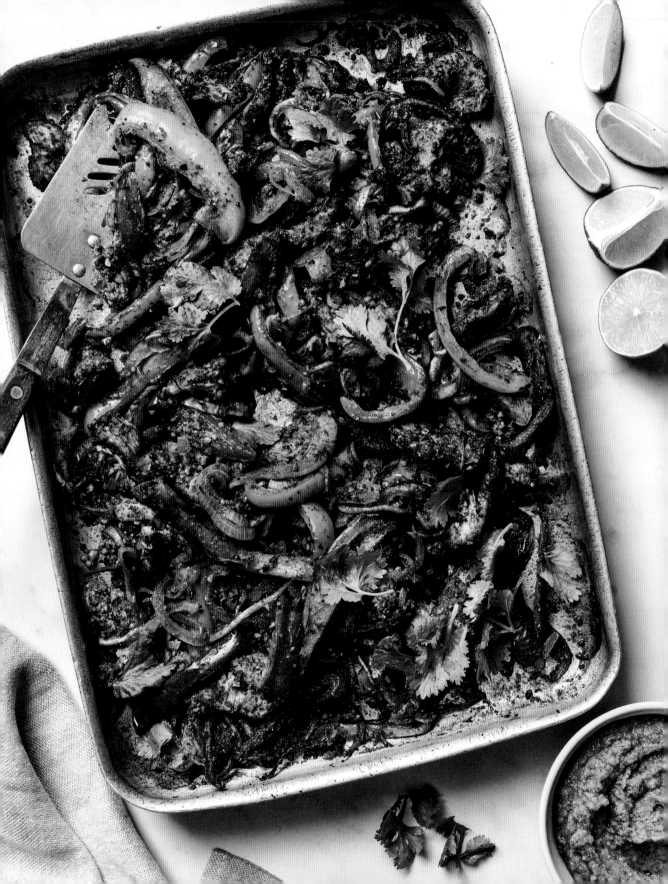

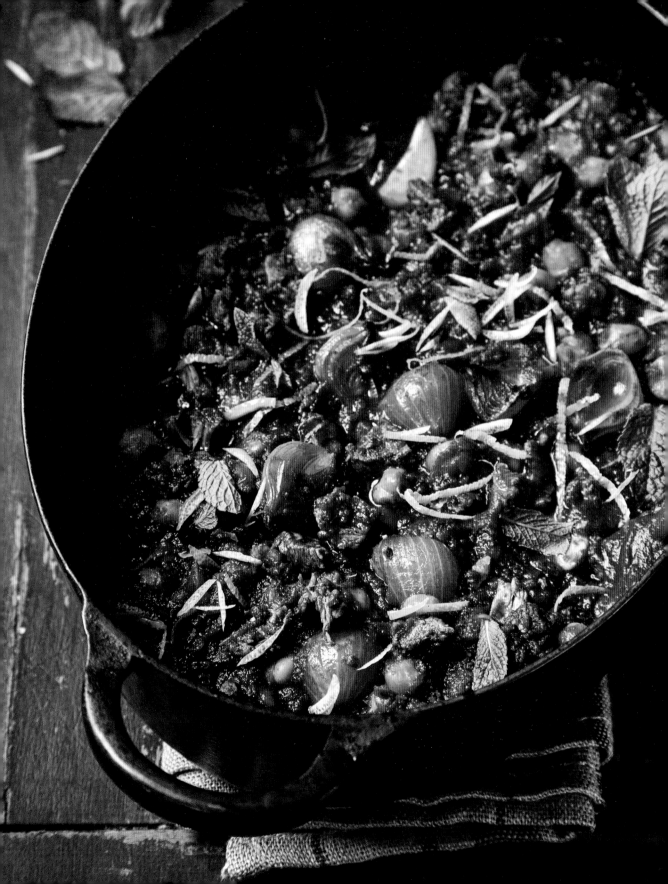

TOMATOEY LAMB & CHICKPEA BAKE

Fibre-rich chickpeas are perfect for adding filling power to a main meal, and the canned variety are so handy for traybakes because they are already cooked and don't require soaking. All the ingredients in this simple traybake are added at the same time, so you can prepare in advance if you have company. Serve with Ribboned Courgette & Zesty Lemon Salad (see page 134), a simple salad or wholemeal pitta bread.

CALORIES PER SERVING: 361

300g (10½oz) lamb neck fillets, chopped small

2 × 400g (14oz) cans chickpeas, drained and rinsed

2 × 400g (14oz) cans chopped tomatoes

3 garlic cloves

finely grated zest and juice of 1 unwaxed lemon

2 tablespoons red wine vinegar

1 tablespoon honey

1 tablespoon paprika

1 teaspoon ground cumin

1 teaspoon salt

6 shallots, peeled and quartered

low-calorie cooking spray

handful of mint leaves

pepper

1. Preheat the oven to 210°C/190°C fan (410°F), Gas Mark 6½.
2. Put the lamb in an ovenproof casserole dish with the chickpeas, tomatoes, garlic, lemon juice, vinegar, honey, paprika, cumin, the salt and some pepper. Mix everything together.
3. Place the shallots on top, then spray with low-calorie cooking spray.
4. Roast for 30 minutes, stir well, then roast for a further 25 minutes.
5. Give a final stir, then scatter with mint leaves and the lemon zest. Serve immediately.

NOTE I try to use lamb neck fillets for this dish, as they are always tender and never chewy. If you can't get hold of neck fillets, you can use diced leg.

GARLICKY MEATBALL PASTA BAKE

When I flat-shared in my 20s I often used to make meatballs with a very rich tomato sauce using lots of olive oil. When I first got my food processor I experimented with whizzing up all of the sauce ingredients together instead and I loved the result. Not only does the flavour of the garlic and chilli really infuse the tomato sauce, but it also saves on chopping and the need for oil. Baked with pasta and melted cheese, this is irresistible. Serve with rocket salad and crunchy sliced sweet red peppers.

CALORIES PER SERVING: 501

500g (1lb 2oz) lean minced beef (less than 5 per cent fat)

low-calorie cooking spray

2 × 400g (14oz) cans chopped tomatoes

5 garlic cloves, peeled

1 whole green chilli, stalk removed

300g (10½oz) dried penne pasta

150g (5½oz) mozzarella

30g (1oz) Parmesan cheese, grated

salt and pepper

TO SERVE
small handful of basil leaves
chopped red chilli (optional)

1. Preheat the oven to 200°C/180°C fan (400°F), Gas Mark 6. Make up the meatballs by simply rolling the minced meat into walnut-sized balls. Fry them over a high heat in a nonstick frying pan with low-calorie cooking spray for 5 minutes, turning them often to brown on all sides.

2. To make the sauce, use a hand blender or a food processor to whizz up the tomatoes, garlic and chilli. Blend until completely smooth, then season with salt and pepper.

3. Transfer the sauce to a saucepan, bring up to a simmer, then add the cooked meatballs.

4. Simmer the sauce and meatballs gently for 30 minutes.

5. Meanwhile, cook the pasta for 12 minutes, drain, then rinse with cold water to prevent it getting sticky.

6. Once the sauce has cooked for 30 minutes, stir the pasta through and spoon it all into an ovenproof dish.

7. Tear up the mozzarella and distribute it evenly over the top, then sprinkle over the Parmesan. Grind some more pepper on top.

8. Bake for 20 minutes until the cheese is golden brown on top. Serve with basil leaves and chopped red chilli (if using).

NOTE If you would like to turn this into a vegetarian meal, have a go at making my Chickpea 'Meatballs' (see page 103) and mix them in with the sauce and pasta.

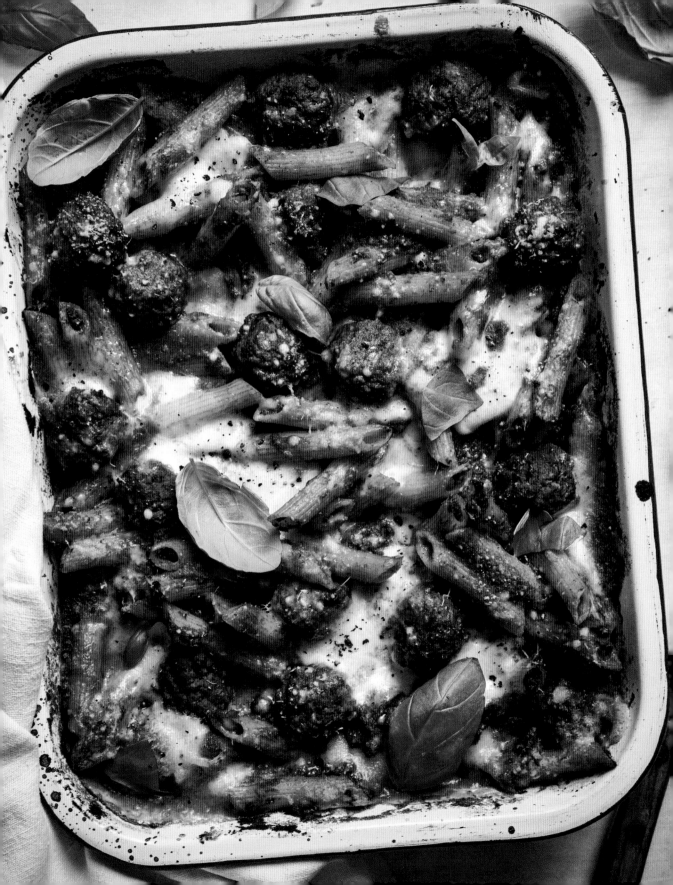

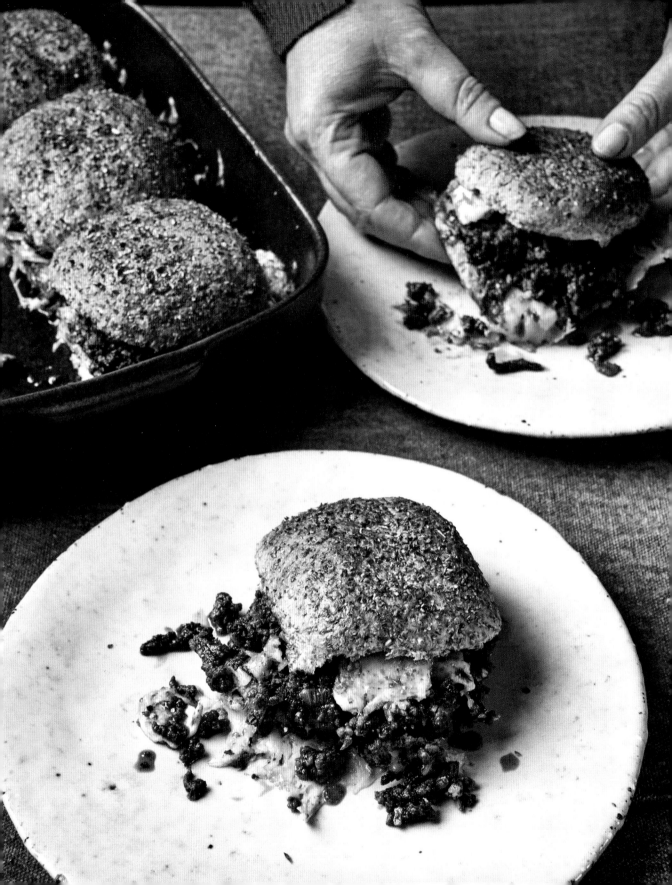

THE CLASSIC SLOPPY JOE
TRAYBAKE STYLE

This rich Bolognese filling, baked in bread rolls with melted cheese, is a fun meal to serve to friends or family. Serve with fries and salad.

CALORIES PER SERVING: 410

500g (1lb 2oz) lean minced beef (less than 5 per cent fat)
1 onion, finely chopped
low-calorie cooking spray
200g (7oz) tomato passata
2 tablespoons tomato purée
1 teaspoon garlic granules
1 teaspoon paprika
1 teaspoon chilli flakes
1 tablespoon Worcestershire sauce
2 teaspoons dried oregano
6 wholemeal bread rolls, sliced in half
125g (4¼oz) Cheddar cheese, grated
100g (3½oz) mozzarella, torn
salt and pepper

1. Preheat the oven to 220°C/200°C fan (425°F), Gas Mark 7.
2. To make the Bolognese sauce, fry the minced beef and onion in low-calorie cooking spray in a large saucepan over a high heat for about 7 minutes until the beef has browned all over.
3. Add the passata, tomato purée, garlic granules, paprika, chilli flakes, Worcestershire sauce and half the oregano, stir, then leave to simmer for 20 minutes. This should end up being quite a dry sauce, to avoid soggy rolls. If it's still a bit wet, increase the heat to high and give it a really good bubble to allow some of the liquid to evaporate.
4. When the meat sauce is nearly ready, layer the bottom half of the sliced bread rolls into the bottom of a casserole dish so they are all lying flat but neatly packed together, and put into the oven for 5 minutes to lightly toast them.
5. Remove the dish from the oven, sprinkle one-third of the Cheddar evenly over the toasted rolls, then spread the Bolognese sauce evenly over the top.
6. Sprinkle the rest of the Cheddar over the top of the Bolognese, then distribute the mozzarella evenly on top.
7. Add the top halves of the bread rolls and squash them down gently onto the cheese. Spray the tops of the rolls with cooking spray and sprinkle over the remaining oregano.
8. Bake on the middle shelf of the oven for 12 minutes until the cheese has melted and the tops of the rolls are toasted.
9. Use a spatula to separate each sloppy joe, then serve.

NOTE If you have Bolognese sauce already in the freezer, you can use it to make this meal even speedier.

PIGGY-IN-THE-MIDDLE

I come back to this recipe again and again because it's simple enough that I can remember the main ingredients off the top of my head, so it's ideal if I'm popping into the supermarket for a quick dinner run! Butter beans are a great source of fibre, protein and iron, and pair really well with sausages. You can serve this alongside a fresh salad or steamed green vegetables, such as green beans or asparagus.

CALORIES PER SERVING: 404

3 small red onions, cut into wedges
1 red pepper, deseeded and sliced
1 yellow pepper, deseeded and sliced
300g (10½oz) cherry tomatoes, halved
6 garlic cloves, peeled but left whole
2 rosemary sprigs
low-calorie cooking spray
8 reduced-fat pork sausages
2 tablespoons balsamic vinegar
1 chicken stock cube
300ml (½ pint) boiling water
1 teaspoon mixed herbs
2 teaspoons wholegrain mustard
2 × 400g (14oz) cans butter beans, drained and rinsed
salt and pepper

1. Preheat the oven to 220°C/200°C fan (425°F), Gas Mark 7.
2. Tumble the onions, peppers, tomatoes, garlic and rosemary into a deep baking tray. Spray with low-calorie cooking spray and stir.
3. Move the vegetables to the edges of the baking tray and line up the sausages in the middle. Prick each sausage a few times with a sharp knife, dress the sausages and vegetables with the balsamic vinegar, then give everything another spray of cooking spray. Place in the oven and roast for 20 minutes.
4. Add the chicken stock cube to the measured boiling water and stir in the mixed herbs and mustard.
5. Remove the tray from the oven, add the butter beans, pour over the stock mixture and give everything a good stir. Turn the sausages over so that the pale sides are showing and season with salt and pepper.
6. Roast for another 20 minutes. The sausages should be browned and the vegetables slightly charred on the edges.

NOTE For extra filling power, you can also roast some new potatoes with this: simply cook them in simmering water for 15 minutes, halve them, then add to the tray with the other vegetables at the start.

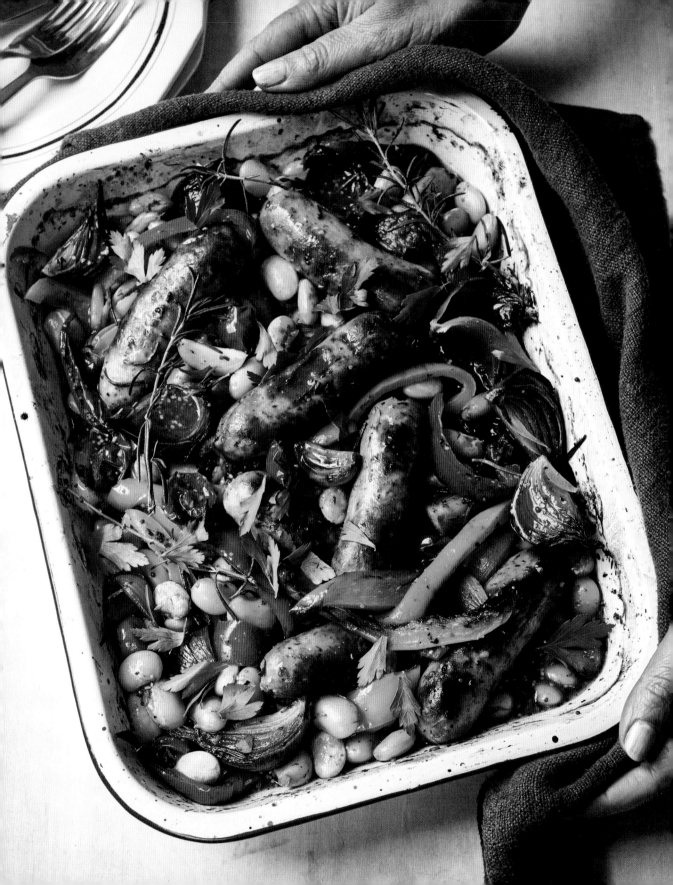

....

FAMILY FAVOURITES

....

• • • • • • • • • • • • •

Regular family mealtimes are not only a chance for quality time,
but a great way to get kids trying new foods, flavours and textures.
Cooking one meal that the whole family will eat is a time saver, plus
it makes it much easier for all of you to stick to those healthier choices,
limiting other temptations.

I know it isn't always easy to find meals that everyone likes, especially if
you have smaller, fussy children. In this chapter are a few of my family's
favourite meals, those that everyone will eat without a murmur, with
some lovely wholesome ingredients mixed in with familiar favourites.

You can get the whole family involved with making these meals –
helping to roll the Crunchy Pea & Mint Fish Bites or the Chickpea
'Meatballs', mashing the potato and butter beans for the Sausage &
Mash Pie or helping to add all the ingredients to the pan for the
Rich & Smoky Veggie Boston Baked Beans. Children usually love to
get involved with the cooking; it's a brilliant way for them to start
to learn important cookery skills that will help them to make
healthy choices in the future.

• • • • • • • • • • • • •

OOZY, CHEESY TOMATO & GNOCCHI BAKE

The gnocchi in this recipe is lovely baked in the oven. It has a satisfying chewy texture and, simmered in rich, herby tomato sauce, then blanketed in melting, oozy mozzarella, it's deliciously simple, one-pot comfort food. Gnocchi can be easily picked up in the fresh pasta section of the supermarket.

CALORIES PER SERVING: 378

1 onion, finely chopped

low-calorie cooking spray

2 garlic cloves, finely chopped

500g (1lb 2oz) tomato passata

1 teaspoon dried oregano, plus extra for sprinkling

10 basil leaves, torn, plus extra to serve

500g (1lb 2oz) pack gnocchi

100g (3½oz) mozzarella, torn up

60g (2¼oz) Cheddar cheese, grated

15g (½oz) Parmesan cheese, grated

salt and pepper

1. Preheat the oven to 220°C/200°C fan (425°F), Gas Mark 7.
2. In a medium-sized ovenproof pot, fry the onion in low-calorie cooking spray for 3–4 minutes until softened.
3. Add the garlic and stir-fry gently for another minute, then add the passata, stirring it through the onions and garlic. Add the oregano and torn basil leaves and season with ¼ teaspoon each of salt and pepper.
4. Stir the gnocchi through the sauce and increase the heat to bring up to a rapid simmer.
5. Remove the dish from the heat, scatter the torn mozzarella evenly over the top, then sprinkle over the Cheddar and Parmesan.
6. Sprinkle with a little more oregano and grind over some pepper.
7. Put the dish into the oven for 15 minutes. When it's ready, the cheese will be golden, bubbling and browning around the edges.
8. Scatter over a few small basil leaves to serve.

NOTE If you fancy adding some extra vegetables to this, then throw in some halved cherry tomatoes or chopped red pepper after the onion, and fry for a few extra minutes before adding the garlic.

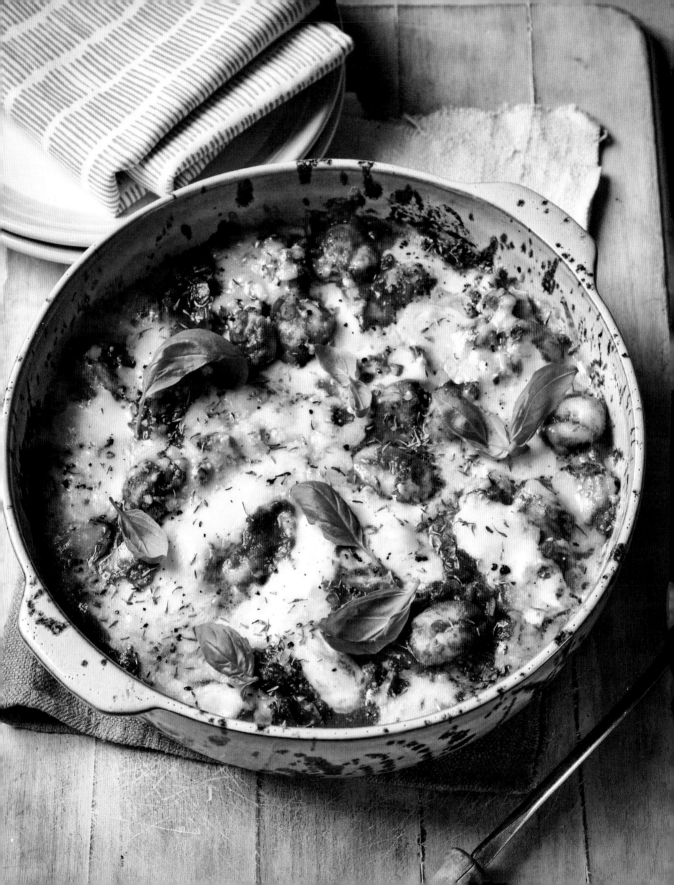

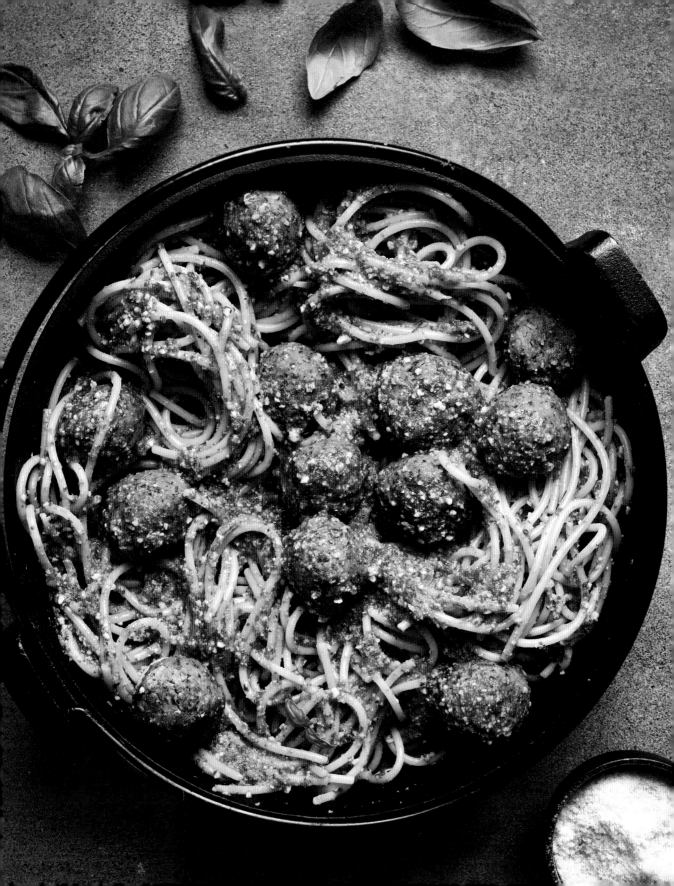

CHICKPEA 'MEATBALLS' & SPAGHETTI

I started making these 'meatballs' for my young daughter, who at one point was finding meat just too chewy, but these are also a great meat-free alternative if you simply want more vegetarian inspiration.

CALORIES PER SERVING: 516

400g (14oz) can chickpeas, drained and rinsed

2 small slices of wholemeal bread, torn into pieces

2 teaspoons Italian seasoning

1 teaspoon onion granules

1 teaspoon garlic granules

10g (¼oz) parsley stalks and leaves

low-calorie cooking spray

4 whole roasted red peppers in brine (about 320g / 11oz), drained

2 garlic cloves, peeled

small handful of basil leaves (about 5g / ⅛oz), plus extra to serve

1 teaspoon dried oregano

60g (2¼oz) blanched almonds

300g (10½oz) wholewheat or regular dried spaghetti

salt and pepper

grated Parmesan, to serve

1. Preheat the oven to 220°C/200°C fan (425°F), Gas Mark 7.
2. Throw the chickpeas into a food processor with the bread, Italian seasoning, onion granules, garlic granules, parsley and some salt and pepper. Pulse in the food processor until everything is blended and starting to clump.
3. Shape the mixture with your hands into 20 small balls. It should be moist enough to hold its shape easily, but if it's too crumbly, whizz a little water into the mixture.
4. Place the balls on a baking tray lined with baking parchment, spray with low-calorie cooking spray and bake for 20 minutes until golden and a little crispy on the outside.
5. Make the sauce by blending the roasted red peppers, garlic, basil, oregano, almonds and some salt and pepper into a smooth sauce.
6. When the meatballs are halfway through their cooking time, cook the spaghetti according to the package instructions.
7. Heat the sauce in a small saucepan, then stir in the baked meatballs. Leave for long enough to heat the sauce through, but do not leave it simmering.
8. Stir the spaghetti through the sauce and serve with Parmesan, torn basil and some more pepper.

NOTE It's easy to make your own roasted peppers. Halve and deseed each pepper. Heat the grill to high and lay the peppers cut-side down on the grill pan. Grill for 15–20 minutes until blackened. Use tongs to place the peppers in a bowl, cover and leave for 30 minutes. The skins should come away easily – rinse them under water to remove the last stubborn bits.

CRUNCHY PEA & MINT FISH BITES

Crunchy on the outside, with a crisp oat and breadcrumb coating, these are a fun way to get a nutritious fish-based meal into the week. Serve with green vegetables, such as broccoli and sugar snap peas, and sweet potato wedges – or try homemade fries (see page 151) – and a wedge of lemon on the side. Any leftovers can easily be frozen for another day.

CALORIES PER SERVING: 150

2 small slices of wholemeal bread
40g (1½oz) oats
400g (14oz) white flaky fish, such as cod, cut into large chunks
100g (3½oz) frozen peas
10 mint leaves
2 eggs
low-calorie cooking spray
salt

TO SERVE
Baked Sweet Potato Wedges (see page 150)
green vegetables of your choice
lemon wedges

1. Preheat the oven to 220°C/200°C fan (425°F), Gas Mark 7.
2. In a food processor, whizz up the bread and oats to form a fine crumb mixture, then empty into a bowl and set aside.
3. Next, use the food processor to make the fish filling. Add the fish, peas and mint into the bowl and pulse to combine. The aim is to break down the fish, but not to purée it.
4. Break the eggs into a bowl and beat them with a fork.
5. Roll the fish into balls that are about 3cm (1¼ inch) in diameter, dip each into the beaten egg, then roll in the breadcrumbs to coat. This mixture should make about 28 balls.
6. Place the prepared balls on a large baking tray lined with baking parchment and sprayed with low-calorie cooking spray. When all the balls have been prepared, spray them with a little more cooking spray and season with salt.
7. Bake on the middle shelf of the oven for 18 minutes. They should be crisp and golden brown on the outside.
8. Serve with sweet potato wedges, green vegetables of your choice and lemon wedges for squeezing over.

NOTE To avoid wasting nearly-out-of-date bread, or ends of loaves, make breadcrumbs with them and pop them into the freezer. These are so handy to have ready for a quick breaded chicken or fish meal, or for making stuffing.

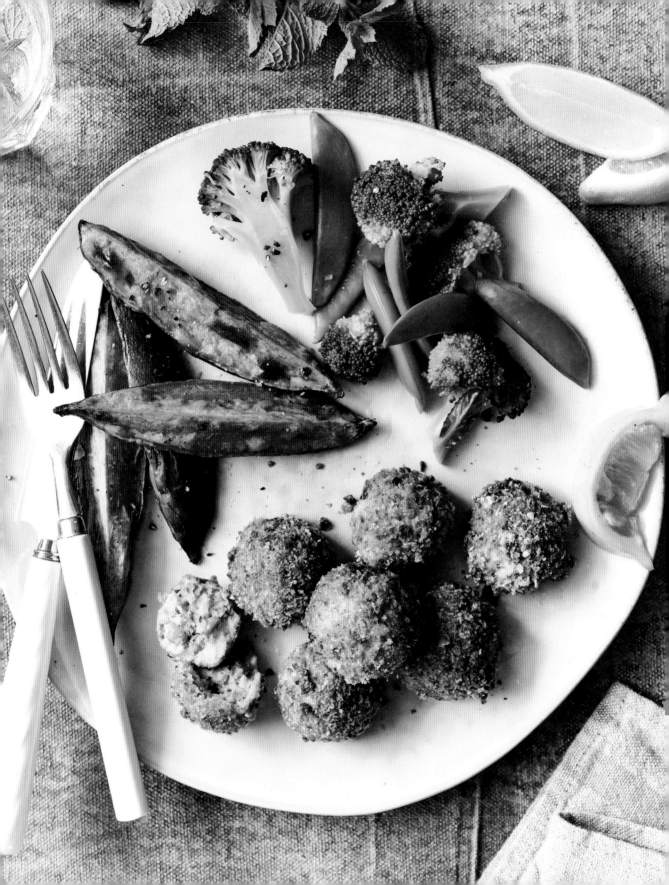

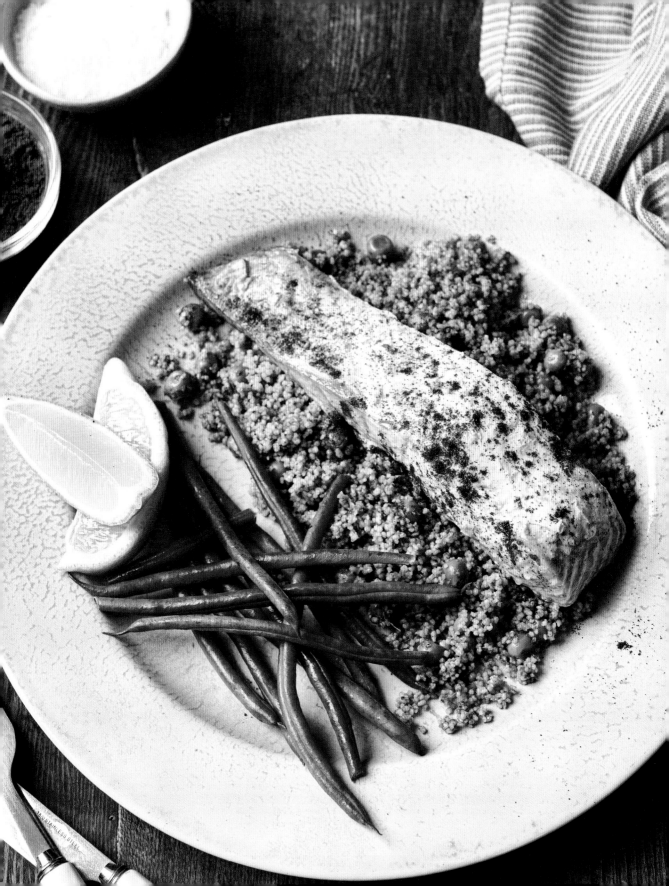

GARLIC & LEMON SALMON
WITH PEA & PESTO COUSCOUS

Ready from start to finish in 20 minutes! Garlic and lemon mayonnaise is brushed over the salmon before roasting, to add amazing flavour and produce perfectly tender fish. The pesto couscous is both delicious and quick to make. Serve with steamed green vegetables or some simple salad leaves.

CALORIES PER SERVING: 547

2 tablespoons light
   mayonnaise
2 garlic cloves, crushed
1 unwaxed lemon
4 salmon fillets
¼ teaspoon paprika
200g (7oz) wholewheat
   couscous
200ml (7fl oz) hot vegetable
   stock
100g (3½oz) frozen peas
3 tablespoons green pesto
salt and pepper
steamed green vegetables of
   your choice, to serve

1. Preheat the oven to 220°C/200°C fan (425°F), Gas Mark 7.
2. In a small bowl, mix the mayonnaise with the crushed garlic. Grate the lemon zest directly over and mix again.
3. Cover a baking tray in foil and place the salmon fillets on top. Using the back of a teaspoon, smear the mayonnaise mixture over the tops and sides of the salmon fillets, then season them with salt and pepper and sprinkle the paprika over the top.
4. Place the salmon on the middle shelf of the oven and roast for 15 minutes.
5. Meanwhile, tip the couscous into a bowl, cover with the hot stock, then cover the bowl with an upturned plate. Leave for 10 minutes. In the meantime, cook the frozen peas according to the package instructions.
6. Fluff the couscous through with a fork, then add the pesto and cooked, drained peas. Mix everything together thoroughly.
7. Divide the couscous between 4 plates and place the salmon on top. Chop the lemon into wedges and serve alongside, with some steamed green vegetables of your choice.

NOTE You can add any seasonal vegetables, such as asparagus, leeks, green beans, courgettes and even Brussels sprouts, to the couscous. Once they're cooked, simply stir them into the couscous with the pesto.

RICH & SMOKY VEGGIE BOSTON BAKED BEANS

Simmered in a sweet and smoky, dark and rich sauce, these are great with a jacket potato or as a toast topping. They also go beautifully alongside a barbecue and always prove a popular dish for a potluck meal.

CALORIES PER SERVING: 226

1 large onion, finely chopped
low-calorie cooking spray
600ml (20fl oz) vegetable stock
3 × 400g (14oz) cans borlotti beans, drained and rinsed
150g (5½oz) tomato passata
1 carrot, peeled and grated
2 tablespoons tomato purée
2 tablespoons maple syrup
2 tablespoons dark soy sauce
1 tablespoon balsamic vinegar
juice of ½ lemon
1 teaspoon smoked paprika
1 teaspoon mustard powder
1 teaspoon garlic granules
1 teaspoon dried thyme
½ teaspoon salt

1. Preheat the oven to 200°C/180°C fan (400°F), Gas Mark 6.
2. In a large, deep pan with a lid, fry the onion in low-calorie cooking spray until soft and lightly browned. Remove from the heat, pour in the stock, then add the rest of the ingredients and give everything a good stir.
3. Pop the lid on the pan and bake in the centre of the oven for 1½ hours. After 1 hour, give the beans a good stir and remove the lid from the pan before cooking for the final 30 minutes.

NOTE If you fancy adding some meat, chopped-up sausage, smoked bacon or pancetta are ideal. Just fry them alongside the onion.

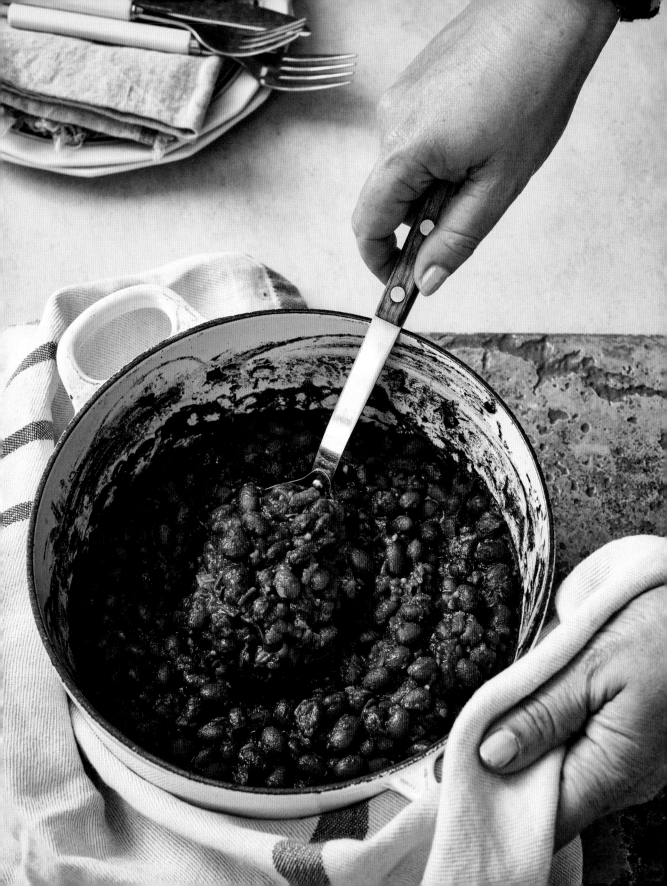

ZA'ATAR & ORANGE ROAST CHICKEN

WITH LEMON ROAST POTATOES

I love to make a Sunday roast with a twist, and finding something that is a little bit different from the norm but that everyone will eat is always a challenge. Za'atar (see page 213) is a Middle-Eastern spice blend that's easy to put together at home but can also be bought as a ready-mixed spice. I love the toasty, herby flavours it adds to chicken. Roast chicken is one of my family's favourites and, cooked in this way, with a hint of orange in the chicken and crispy, lemony potatoes (see photograph on pages 112–13), I am always left with clean plates.

CALORIES PER SERVING: 466

FOR THE CHICKEN
1 small orange
1 whole chicken
1 tablespoon Za'atar (see page 213)
low-calorie cooking spray

FOR THE POTATOES
1kg (2lb 4oz) potatoes, peeled and halved
50ml (2fl oz) chicken stock
1 large unwaxed lemon
1 garlic bulb, cloves separated but skins left on
salt and pepper

1. Preheat the oven to 200°C/180°C fan (400°F), Gas Mark 6.
2. Prick the orange all over with a sharp knife and insert into the chicken's cavity. Place the chicken in a roasting tin, sprinkle the Za'atar spice mix over the skin, then spray all over with low-calorie cooking spray. Cover with foil and place on the middle shelf of the oven for 1 hour.
3. While the chicken starts to cook, prepare the potatoes. Put them in a large saucepan, cover with cold water, place a lid on the pan, set over a high heat and bring to the boil. Once boiling, reduce the temperature to a gentle simmer and cook for 10 minutes, until a little bit soft on the outside. Drain off the water, then shake in the pan with the lid on to roughen up the outsides (the key to lovely crispy potatoes).
4. While the parboiled potatoes are still in the pan, pour the chicken stock over them, then grate the zest of the lemon over and add a few grinds of salt and pepper. Stir the potatoes around until thoroughly coated, then spray them with cooking spray.

5. Spray a baking tray with cooking spray and add the potatoes and garlic cloves. Quarter the lemon and add the wedges to the pan. Then spray all over once more with cooking spray.

6. After the chicken has been cooking for 1 hour, increase the oven temperature to 220°C/200°C fan (425°F), Gas Mark 7, and put the tray of potatoes in to cook. They will take 45 minutes and need to be turned halfway through. Remove the foil from the chicken and return it to the oven for about 30 minutes, depending on the size of the bird.

7. When the chicken is cooked (see note, below), remove it from the oven, cover it with the foil and allow it to rest for 15 minutes while the potatoes finish cooking.

8. Serve with your favourite vegetables.

NOTE Remove the uncooked chicken from the refrigerator and allow it to sit at room temperature for at least 30 minutes before cooking. To calculate the cooking time for a whole chicken, allow 20 minutes per 450g (1lb), plus an extra 15–20 minutes. A meat thermometer can be really helpful if you aren't confident about knowing when the chicken is done.

> **ALWAYS REST A ROAST CHICKEN FOR AT LEAST 15 MINUTES AFTER COOKING TO KEEP THE JUICES IN AND THE MEAT SUCCULENT. GET THE MOST OUT OF YOUR CHICKEN BY MAKING A STOCK WITH THE LEFTOVERS (SEE PAGE 217).**

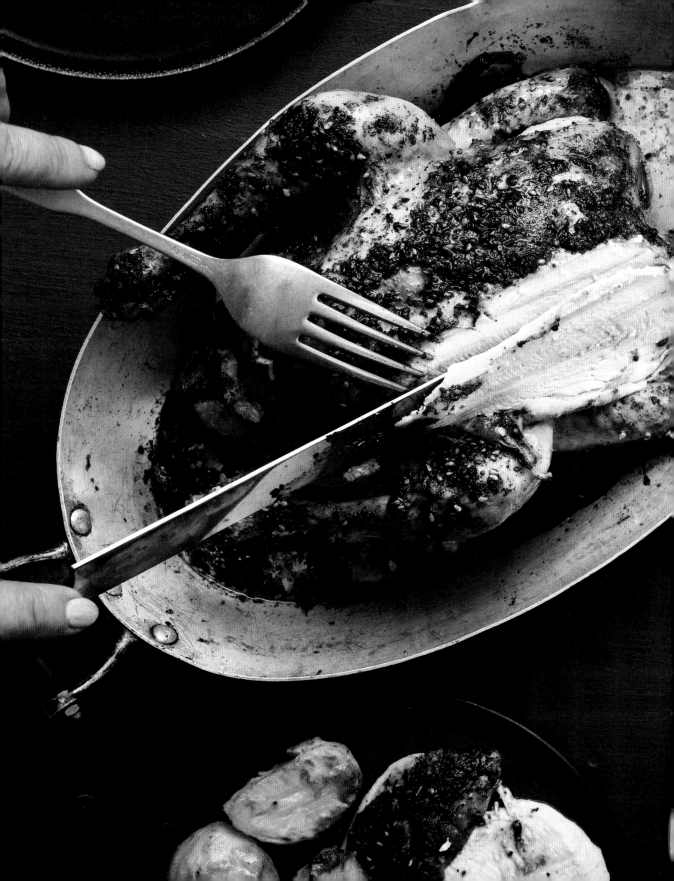

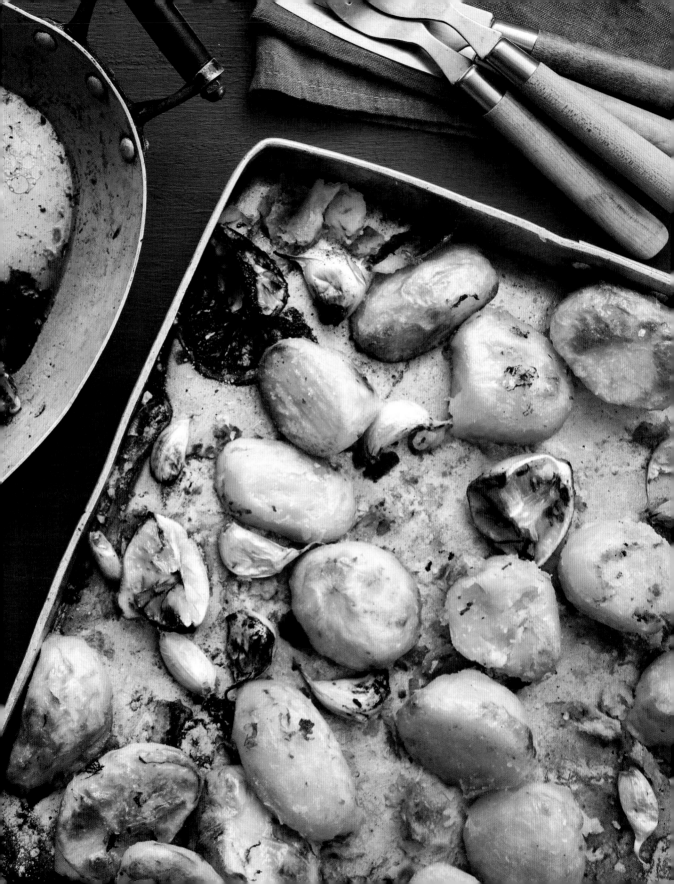

LEMONY CHICKEN & COURGETTE CARBONARA

This is a really lovely light, summery pasta. The creamy, garlicky carbonara has just a hint of lemon. It is a brilliant way to use up in-season courgettes, which I think are best eaten with the fresh crunch that they have when eaten raw or when only very lightly cooked.

CALORIES PER SERVING: 442

240g (8½oz) dried spaghetti

4 egg yolks

60g (2¼oz) Parmesan cheese, finely grated

2 chicken breasts, chopped small

low-calorie cooking spray

4 garlic cloves, crushed

finely grated zest and juice of 2 unwaxed lemons

2 courgettes (about 250g / 9oz), sliced into 3mm (⅛ inch) pieces, then halved

salt and pepper

handful of parsley leaves, finely chopped, to serve

1. Put the spaghetti in a large pan of boiling water to simmer for 11 minutes.
2. Beat the egg yolks in a medium-sized bowl, then beat in the Parmesan.
3. Meanwhile, in a large frying pan or sauté pan, fry the chicken over a high heat in low-calorie cooking spray until no pink is showing (about 3 minutes), then add the garlic, lemon zest and juice, and season with salt and pepper. Keep frying gently while the spaghetti is cooking.
4. When the pasta is nearly ready, take a ladleful of the pasta water, add it to the egg mixture and mix it in thoroughly.
5. Stir the courgette pieces in with the chicken.
6. Check the spaghetti is cooked, then drain it.
7. Remove the pan of chicken and courgette from the heat, add the spaghetti and then the egg mixture. Stir well until everything is coated with the sauce. Serve with chopped parsley and grind more pepper over.

NOTE You can swap the chicken for bacon and leave out the lemon juice and zest for a more traditional carbonara. Why not whip up the leftover egg whites to make some crunchy crumble topping (see page 193) to go in the freezer ready for the next time you make crumble?

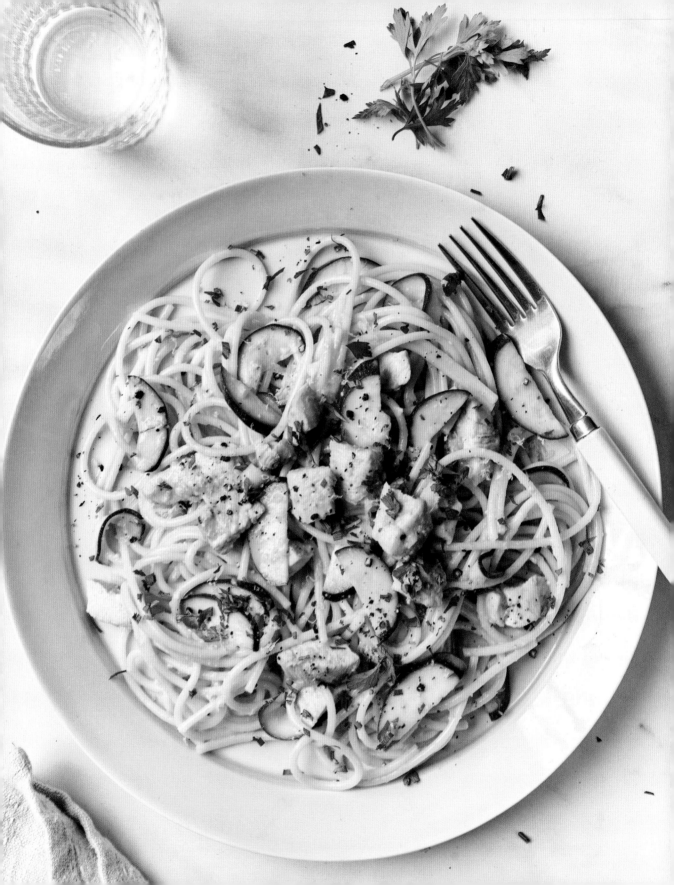

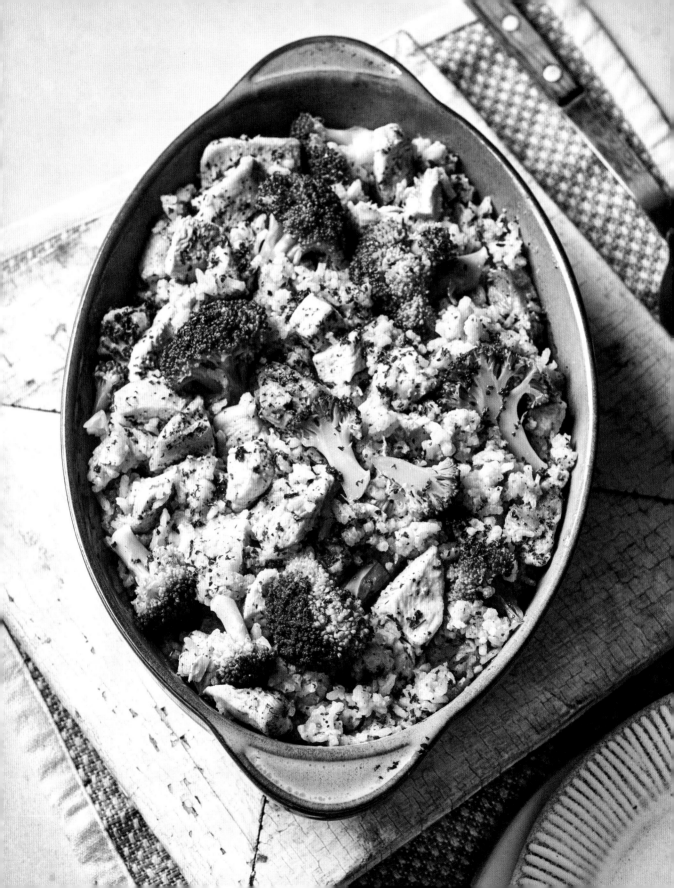

SIMPLE OVEN-BAKED CHICKEN & BROCCOLI RICE

A simple but tasty dish that involves very little preparation or hands-on time and few ingredients. This savoury rice has a subtle herby flavour and is the perfect one-pot dinner at the end of a busy day.

CALORIES PER SERVING: 429

3 chicken breasts, chopped
2 teaspoons dried parsley
1 teaspoon garlic granules
1 teaspoon onion granules
½ teaspoon salt
¼ teaspoon pepper
low-calorie cooking spray
250g (9oz) long-grain rice
650ml (1 pint 2½fl oz) hot chicken stock
1 head of broccoli (about 200g / 7oz), broken into florets

1. Preheat the oven to 220°C/200°C fan (425°F), Gas Mark 7.
2. In a large ovenproof dish, mix the chicken with the dried parsley, garlic granules, onion granules and salt and pepper. Spray with low-calorie cooking spray, then mix in the rice.
3. Pour the hot stock over the rice, ensure everything is submerged, then cover the dish tightly with foil.
4. Bake on the middle shelf of the oven for 30 minutes.
5. Remove the dish from the oven, fluff up the rice with a fork, then scatter the broccoli over the top in a single layer.
6. Replace the foil lid and cook in the oven for a further 15 minutes. By this time the stock should have been absorbed, the rice will be fluffy and cooked through, and the broccoli perfectly steamed. If the rice still has a bit of bite, put it back in the oven until it is fully cooked through.

NOTE This is a nice easy dish to jazz up with everyone's favourite vegetables for any fussy eaters. Try adding peas, green beans, cauliflower or asparagus. If you fancy a little more flavour, add the finely grated zest and juice of an unwaxed lemon when you mix up the raw chicken and spices.

SAUSAGE & MASH PIE

I've always been a big fan of sausage, mash and gravy, and this pie includes all these elements. With butter beans mashed into the potatoes and lentils cooked in with the gravy, this is an excellent fibre boost with great filling power. Serve with your favourite green vegetables.

CALORIES PER SERVING: 497

2 red onions, finely chopped
low-calorie cooking spray
1 garlic clove, crushed
8 reduced-fat pork sausages, each sliced into 6 pieces
250ml (9fl oz) beef stock
390g (13½oz) can green lentils, drained and rinsed
2 tablespoons tomato purée
1 teaspoon dried thyme
1 tablespoon brown sauce
3–4 white potatoes (total weight 700g / 1lb 9oz), peeled and cut into chunks
400g (14oz) can butter beans, drained and rinsed
4 tablespoons semi-skimmed milk
salt and pepper

1. Preheat the oven to 220°C/200°C fan (425°F), Gas Mark 7.
2. In a sauté pan, fry the onions gently in low-calorie cooking spray for about 6 minutes, until they are starting to soften.
3. Add the garlic and stir-fry for 30 seconds, then add the chopped-up sausages. Increase the heat and stir-fry for about 5 minutes, until the sausages are starting to brown.
4. Pour in the stock, add the lentils, tomato purée, thyme and brown sauce and season with salt and pepper. Allow to simmer gently over a low heat while you cook the potatoes.
5. In a medium-sized saucepan, cover the potato chunks with boiling water, bring to the boil, then simmer for 10 minutes. After this time, add the butter beans to the potatoes and simmer for another 10 minutes.
6. Drain the potatoes and butterbeans and, using a potato masher, mash them into a creamy, smooth mash with the milk. Season with a little salt and pepper.
7. Spoon the sausage mixture into an ovenproof dish, then spread the mashed potato evenly over the top. Use a fork to rough up the top of the potato by dragging it vertically and then horizontally over the potato, creating a criss-cross pattern that will give some lovely crispy bits when baked.
8. Spray the top of the pie with some cooking spray, then bake for 25–30 minutes until golden brown, with some crispy edges on top. Serve with your favourite vegetables.

NOTE Lots of different vegetables can be added to the sauce – leeks and celery can be fried at the same time as the sausages, or diced carrots or sweet potato added with the stock.

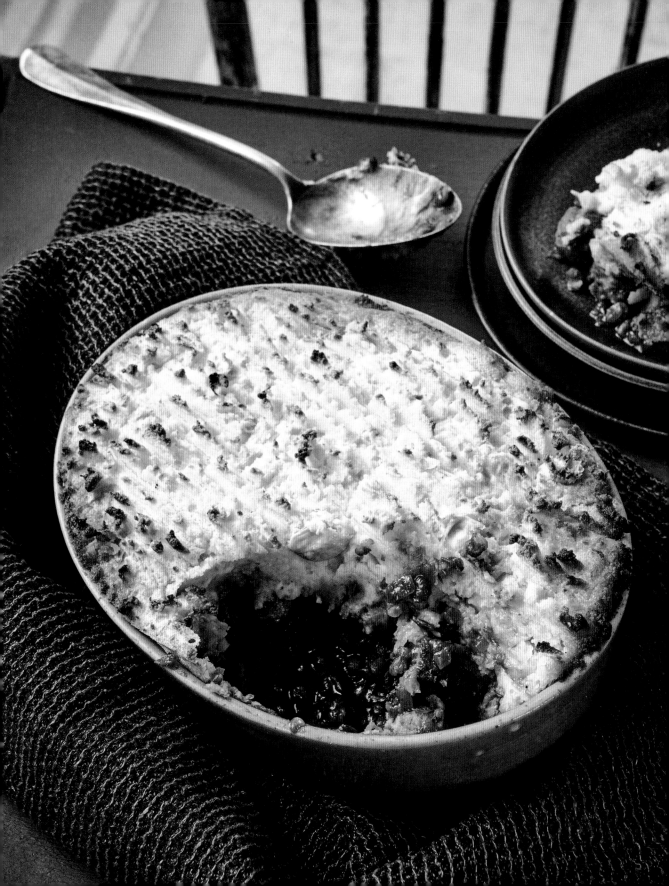

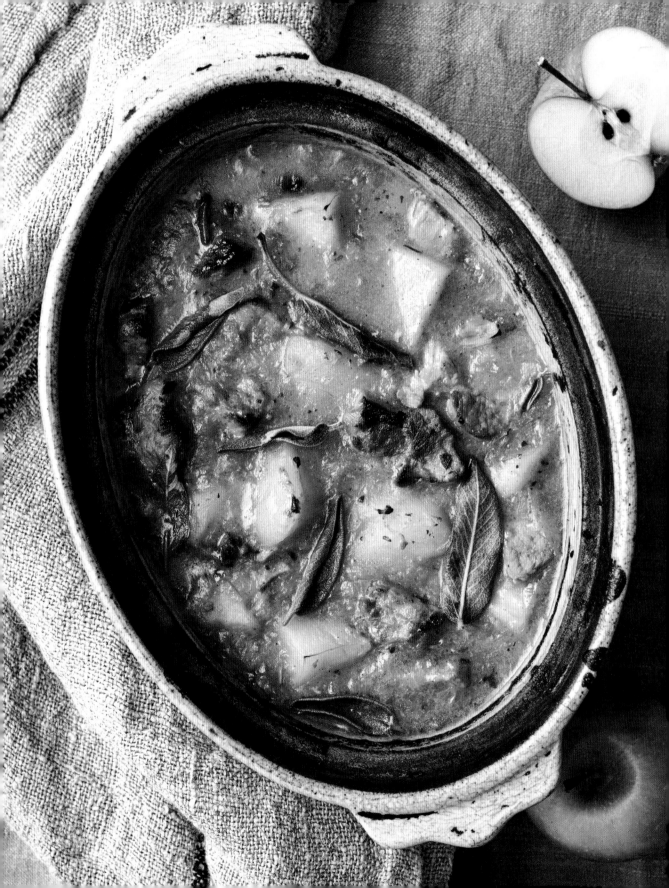

RUSTIC DEVONSHIRE PORK IN CIDER

This is a childhood favourite of mine, one that my Grandma and Mum would often cook, and the first dish in which I (finally) consented to eat onions! The flavours are simple, but the result is warming, comforting and satisfying. It's also a great seasonal all-rounder, working as both a summer and a winter casserole. I add potatoes to save having to make a separate side dish, but I always try to serve it alongside green vegetables such as peas or broccoli.

CALORIES PER SERVING: 479

1 teaspoon butter

3 onions, finely chopped

500g (1lb 2oz) pork loin steaks, fat trimmed away, chopped

6 sage leaves, finely chopped, plus a few more leaves, torn, to serve

2 apples, peeled and finely chopped

250ml (9fl oz) cider

700g (1lb 9oz) potatoes, peeled and cut into chunks

1 teaspoon Dijon mustard

500ml (18fl oz) hot chicken stock

salt and pepper

1. Preheat the oven to 200°C/180°C fan (400°F), Gas Mark 6.
2. Melt the butter in a large casserole dish and fry the onions for 10 minutes, until softened and lightly golden.
3. Add the pork, sage and apples and stir-fry over a high heat for 2 minutes.
4. Pour in the cider, bring to the boil, then add the potatoes, mustard and stock. Season with salt and pepper. Stir everything together, place a lid on the pan and bake in the oven for 45 minutes.
5. Remove the lid and bake for another 15 minutes.
6. Scatter with torn sage leaves and grind over a little more pepper to serve.

NOTE This is delicious even with cheap cider, but using local cider can add depth of flavour. If you'd like to make this in a slow cooker, pre-fry the onions and put them in the slow cooker bowl with all the ingredients except the potatoes. Cook on high for 6–8 hours, or low for 10–12 hours. Add the potato chunks 1 hour before the end of the cooking time.

POT-ROAST BEEF BRISKET
WITH HASSELBACK CARROTS

This fall-apart tender beef, cooked in a rich, flavourful gravy, will scent the house with the most amazing aromas while it's cooking.

CALORIES PER SERVING: 341

low-calorie cooking spray

1kg (2lb 4oz) rolled beef brisket

2 red onions, finely chopped

2 garlic cloves, crushed

2 celery sticks

1 litre (1¾ pints) beef stock

1 teaspoon mustard powder

1 tablespoon Worcestershire sauce

1 teaspoon dried thyme

1 teaspoon dried rosemary

1 tablespoon tomato purée

2 teaspoons cornflour

8 similar-sized carrots, peeled but left whole

salt and pepper

1. Preheat the oven to 170°C/150°C fan (340°F), Gas Mark 3½.

2. Spray a frying pan with low-calorie cooking spray and sear the beef over a high heat for 1 minute on each side.

3. Transfer the beef to a casserole dish, then put the onions, garlic and celery into the frying pan and stir-fry for 5 minutes. Transfer these to the casserole dish.

4. Pour the beef stock into a jug and add the mustard powder, Worcestershire sauce, thyme, rosemary and tomato purée. Mix everything together. In a small dish, mix 1 tablespoon cold water with the cornflour and stir until smooth. Pour this into the stock.

5. Pour the stock over the beef and season with salt and pepper. Cover with a lid and cook in the oven for 4 hours, turning the meat once halfway through the cooking time.

6. When the beef only has 1 hour or so left to cook, prepare the carrots. Boil them whole for 10 minutes, then drain and cool them by running under cold water.

7. Place each carrot lengthways in parallel between the handles of two wooden spoons and, using a sharp knife, slice evenly across each carrot, with intervals of about 5mm (¼ inch) between each cut.

8. Place the carrots on a baking tray, spray with cooking spray and season with salt and pepper. Roast for 40 minutes, until browned and very tender.

9. When the beef is cooked, remove the beef from the dish and use a hand blender to whizz up the remaining contents of the pan into a velvety gravy.

10. Either slice the beef finely or pull it apart with 2 forks. Serve with the gravy and the hasselback carrots.

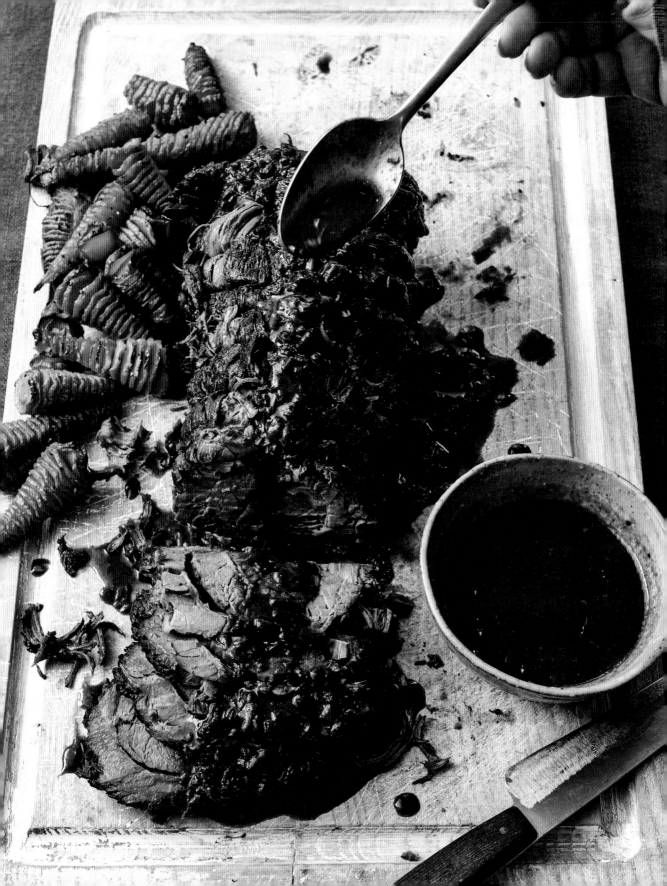

LIGHT DISHES & SIDES

• • • • • • • • • • • • •

It's really useful to have some quick and easy side dish ideas up your sleeve, so you can make sure you get a good portion of vegetables with every meal. There are some brilliant ways to pre-prepare them, so you can easily add extra veg to meals.

My Baked Sweet Potato Falafel is one of my most popular blog recipes – they are a great healthy snack, or serve them with salad for a quick lunch.

I like to make up a big batch of Chilli Roasted Vegetables, which I keep in an airtight container in the refrigerator for up to 5 days. These work with lots of main meals, warm or cold, or can be used alongside leftover meat or a jacket potato for a quick lunch option. Pickling is a really good idea for using up veg that might otherwise go to waste and gives it a new lease of life, and pickles such as Snappy Quick-pickled Carrots can be stored ready to be served up when you need them.

A hearty salad with a tasty dressing is perfect for taking over to a friend's barbecue or made up in advance for easy lunches for work or home: try the Zingy Shredded Thai Chicken, Carrot & Red Cabbage Salad or the Smoked Mackerel Salad with Garlic Aïoli.

• • • • • • • • • • • • •

5-VEG ONION BHAJI CRUST QUICHE

A traditional quiche often contains cream and cheese with a buttery pastry case. With some easy changes – a quinoa crust, spices and lots of vegetables – you can make a delicious quiche, full of goodness.

CALORIES PER SERVING: 200

60g (2¼oz) quinoa

250ml (9fl oz) water

2 small onions, halved and sliced

1 carrot, peeled and grated (about 100g / 3½oz)

1 teaspoon ground turmeric

1 teaspoon garam masala

1 teaspoon cumin seeds, plus more to serve

½ teaspoon chilli powder

5 eggs

low-calorie cooking spray

50ml (2fl oz) semi-skimmed milk

1 roasted red pepper in brine, drained and finely chopped

30g (1oz) baby spinach, roughly chopped

50g (1¾oz) frozen peas

salt and pepper

handful of coriander leaves, to serve

1. Preheat the oven to 220°C/200°C fan (425°F), Gas Mark 7.
2. Tip the quinoa into a small saucepan, cover with the measured cold water and bring to the boil. Add the onions and simmer gently for 12 minutes, until all the water has been absorbed and the grains have swollen. Spoon the quinoa and onions into a mixing bowl and allow to cool for 10 minutes.
3. Add the carrot, then stir in the turmeric, garam masala, cumin seeds and chilli powder. Season with salt and pepper.
4. Take one of the eggs and separate the white from the yolk. Stir the egg white through the quinoa mixture.
5. Spray a 24cm (9½ inch) tart tin with a solid base with low-calorie cooking spray, then add the quinoa mixture. Pat it down into the dish, spreading it evenly to cover the base and sides and using a metal spoon to pack it in and shape it to the dish.
6. Spray the quinoa with cooking spray again, then bake on the top shelf of the oven for 20 minutes, until the crust is golden and browning on the edges.
7. While the crust is cooking, beat the 4 remaining eggs with the leftover yolk, add the milk, then stir in the red pepper, spinach and peas. Season with salt and pepper.
8. Remove the crust from the oven and reduce the oven temperature to 180°C/160°C fan (350°F), Gas Mark 4. Pour the egg mixture into the crust, return it to the oven and cook for 25 minutes. Serve warm or cold, scattered with cumin seeds and sprinkled with coriander.

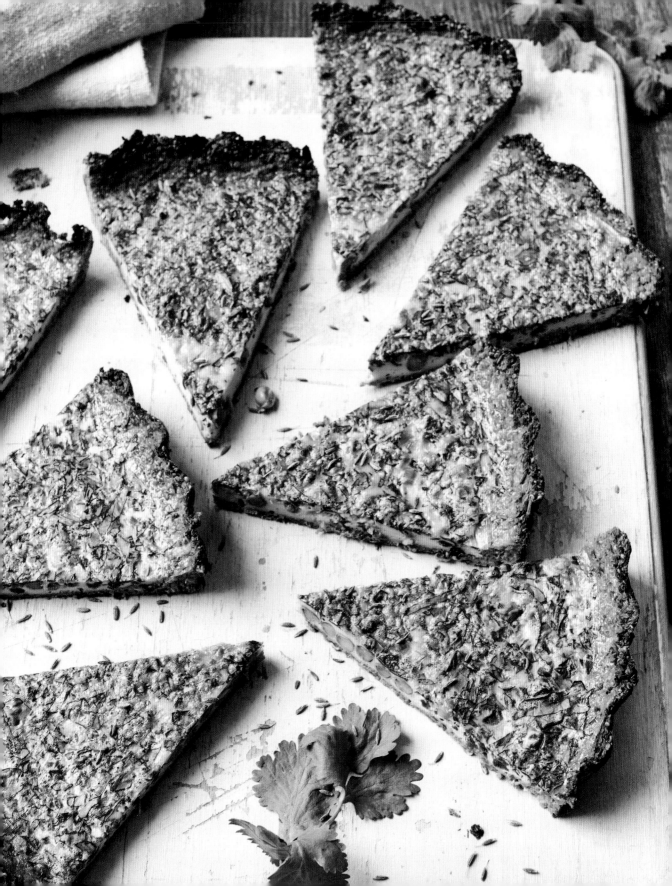

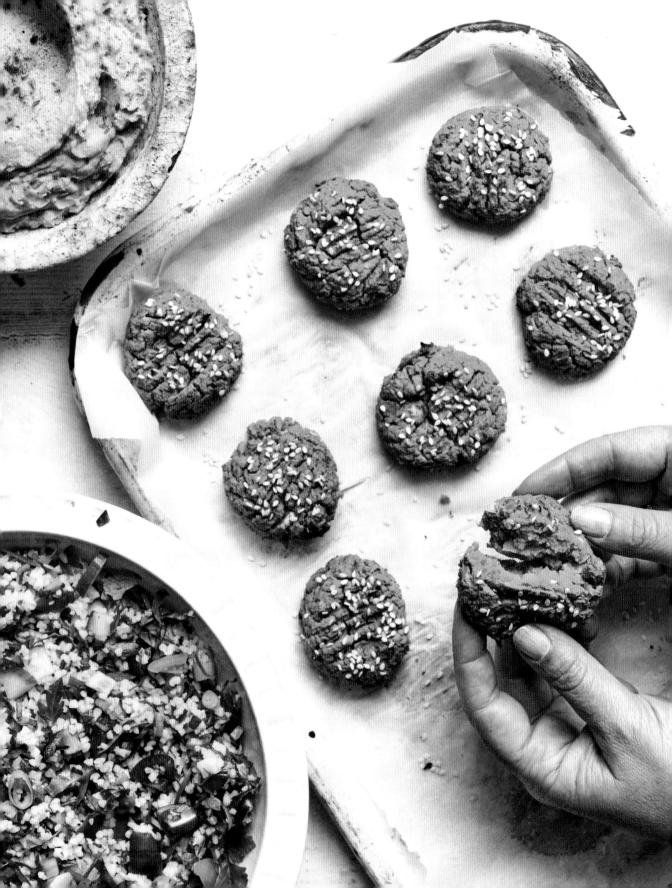

BAKED SWEET POTATO FALAFEL

The sweet potato gives a moist centre to these falafel, which are a great alternative to the traditional deep-fried version, though these bite-sized mouthfuls still carry the classic flavours of cumin, coriander and garlic. With the filling power of chickpeas, they make a great snack or salad accompaniment. I usually serve them with Table-top Tabbouleh (see page 133) and hummus.

CALORIES PER SERVING: 131

2 small sweet potatoes, or 1 large one
400g (14oz) can chickpeas, drained and rinsed
2 garlic cloves, peeled
1½ teaspoons ground cumin
1½ teaspoons ground coriander
juice of ½ lemon
low-calorie cooking spray
sesame seeds (optional)
salt and pepper

1. Either bake or microwave the sweet potatoes so the flesh is soft and fudgy. To microwave, pierce the skin a few times, pop on a microwaveable plate and cook for 5–8 minutes until cooked through. To bake, preheat the oven to 200°C/180°C fan (400°F), Gas Mark 6. Prick the potatoes a few times with a sharp knife and place them on a baking tray lined with foil. Bake for 40–45 minutes until they are tender throughout.

2. Allow the sweet potatoes to cool enough to handle, then scoop out the flesh and put it, along with all the other ingredients, apart from the low-calorie cooking spray and sesame seeds, into a food processor, seasoning to taste. Whizz up until completely blended.

3. Line a baking tray with baking parchment and spray with cooking spray. Use your hands to shape the mixture into small rounds. Press down gently on each with a fork to flatten slightly and leave its imprint. If you want to use the sesame seeds, sprinkle a couple of pinches over the top now.

4. Bake in the oven for 25 minutes, until the outsides are firm and the bottoms are crispy.

NOTE You can make spicy falafel by adding ½ teaspoon chilli powder or some finely chopped fresh chilli. Keep the falafel in an airtight container in the refrigerator for up to 5 days or freeze them for when you need them.

BUFFALO ROASTED CHICKPEAS

Crunchy on the outside, chewy on the inside, these smoky, chilli-infused roasted chickpeas are temptingly moreish both hot and cold. They make a great snack on their own or add a tasty and healthy crunch sprinkled over a salad or soup instead of croutons.

**CALORIES PER
SERVING: 103**

2 × 400g (14oz) cans
   chickpeas, drained and
   rinsed
1 tablespoon hot chilli sauce,
   such as sriracha
1 teaspoon smoked paprika
1 teaspoon garlic granules
low-calorie cooking spray
1 teaspoon freshly ground
   salt

1. Preheat the oven to 220°C/200°C fan (425°F), Gas Mark 7.
2. Mix the chickpeas with the chilli sauce, smoked paprika and garlic granules, then spray them with low-calorie cooking spray.
3. Line a baking tray with baking parchment and spread the chickpeas out evenly in a single layer.
4. Spray again with cooking spray, sprinkle over the salt and bake in the oven for 30 minutes. Halfway through the cooking time, give them a shake so they cook evenly.
5. When they are done they will be a dark roasted colour, but not burnt. Remove them from the oven and leave them out for 10 minutes, as they crisp up a little more as they steam.

NOTE If you don't eat these all at once (though that's unheard of in my house), they will keep in an airtight container for up to 4 days.

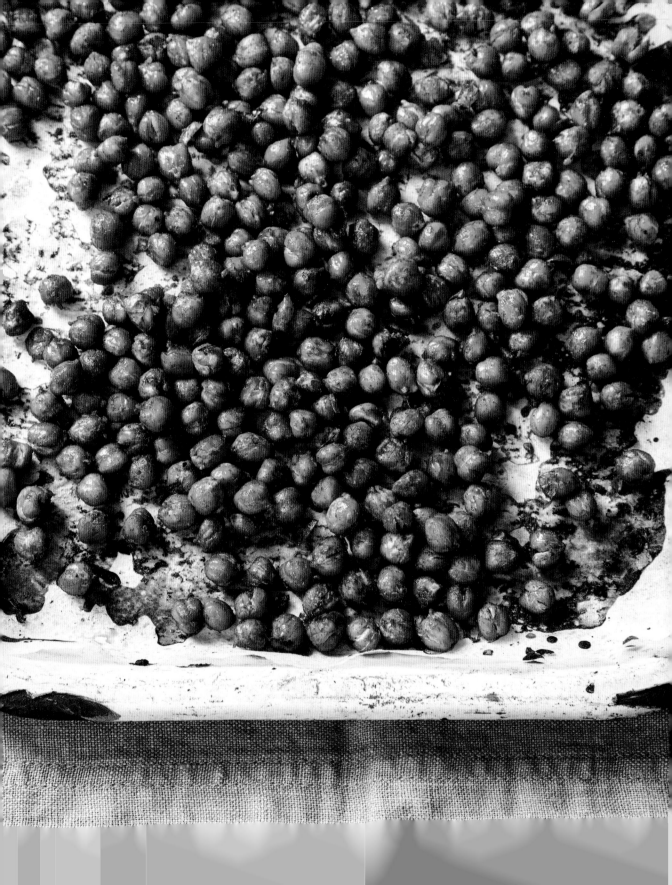

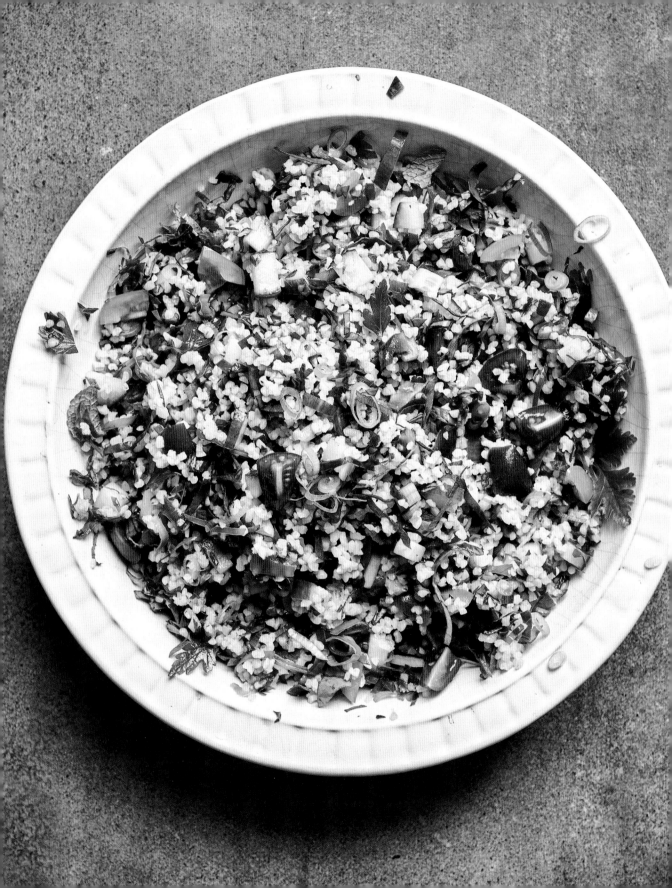

TABLE-TOP TABBOULEH

This dish is inspired by the Middle Eastern tabbouleh salad – fresh, herby and satisfying, with a hint of garlic and lemon and fresh bursts of tomato and cucumber. An easy lunch or dinner, it is a great dish to scale up. If I am catering for a crowd, I will often make a big batch of this and serve it up on a huge platter. Serve this with salty grilled halloumi and rocket or Gently Spiced Sweet Potato Hummus (see page 206) and Baked Sweet Potato Falafel (see page 129).

CALORIES PER SERVING: 193

200g (7oz) bulgur wheat
450ml (16fl oz) boiling water
4 spring onions, trimmed and finely sliced
100g (3½oz) cherry tomatoes, finely chopped
50g (1¾oz) baby spinach, finely chopped
100g (3½oz) cucumber, finely chopped
1 garlic clove, crushed
10g (¼oz) parsley leaves, finely chopped
10g (¼oz) mint leaves, finely chopped
½ teaspoon salt
juice of 1 lemon

1. Pour the bulgur wheat and measured water into a small saucepan, bring it to a simmer, cover with a lid and allow it to simmer gently for about 12 minutes, until tender.

2. Remove it from the heat, fluff it through with a fork, then cover again and leave to rest for 10 minutes. (Either prepare this in advance to allow it time to cool or spread it on to a baking tray after cooking so it cools quickly, before adding it to the other ingredients.)

3. Put the spring onions in a large bowl with the tomatoes, spinach, cucumber, garlic, parsley, mint and salt, and give everything a good stir.

4. Add the cooled bulgur wheat, dress with the lemon juice and mix everything together thoroughly.

NOTE This is a great base for any fresh, seasonal vegetables that you have in. Try it with sugarsnap peas, green beans, broad beans, courgettes, carrots and even chillies. It's a great way to use up leftover vegetables.

RIBBONED COURGETTE & ZESTY LEMON SALAD

The simplest of salads, this takes just minutes to put together but it's one of my favourite ways to eat courgette – served raw and with a slight bite. This makes a great complement to so many meals. I like to serve it with Lightning-quick Tuna, Chilli & Cannellini Bean Linguine, Sumac Chicken, Potato & Cauliflower and Tomatoey Lamb & Chickpea Bake (see pages 48, 87 and 91). It really is one of the most versatile side dishes!

CALORIES PER SERVING: 13

2–3 (about 300g / 10½oz) courgettes
juice of ½ lemon
sea salt flakes

1. Using a y-shaped peeler, strip the courgettes lengthways into thin ribbons by working your way around the courgette in a circular motion. I take about 3 strips from each section before moving around to the next part, depending on the size of the courgette. Leave behind most of the seedy centres.
2. Place the courgette ribbons in a bowl, dress with the lemon juice and grind some salt coarsely over the top. Use your hands to toss the courgette ribbons in the dressing and serve immediately.

NOTE If you want to give this a bit of a kick, add some chopped fresh chilli – red chilli will really stand out against the vibrant green of the courgettes.

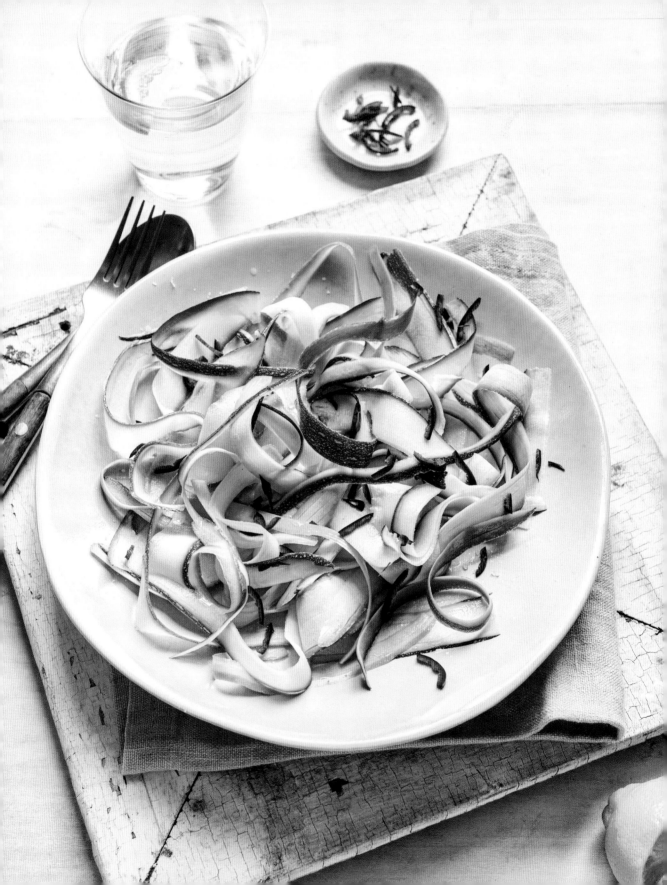

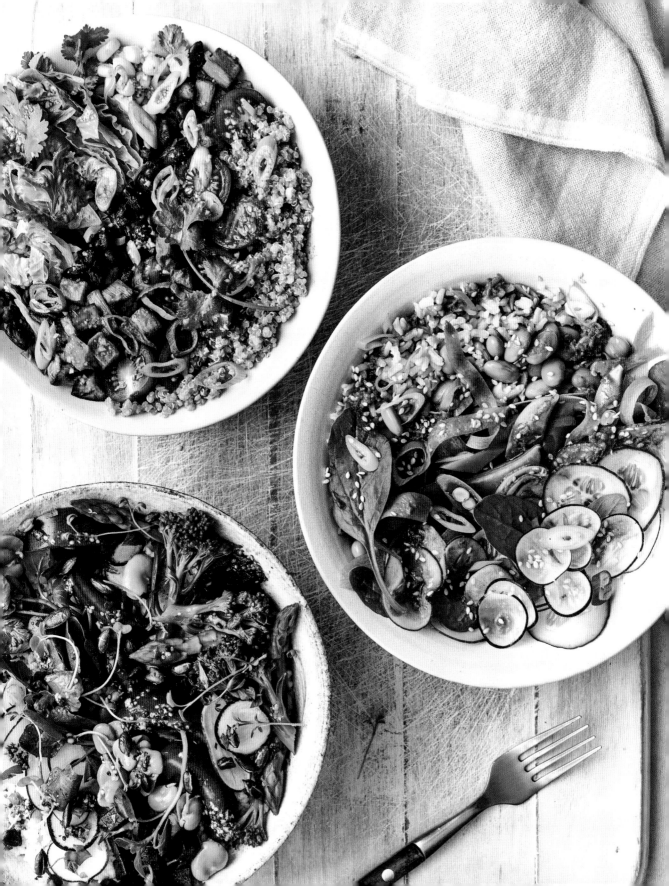

MEXICAN-STYLE BOUNTY BOWL

'Bounty bowls' are bowls filled to the brim with nourishing ingredients and lots of choice. They not only look beautiful, but are filling, tasty and full of wholesome goodness. Usually a base grain and salad is dressed up with a variety of vegetables, then a tasty dressing is added. I've created three ideas here, but you can really be as imaginative as you like with what goes in and how you dress it. And remember: making it look pretty is half the fun!

CALORIES PER SERVING: 299

---

1 medium sweet potato, peeled and cut into small cubes

low-calorie cooking spray

80g (2¾oz) quinoa

8 cherry tomatoes, halved

80g (2¾oz) frozen sweetcorn, cooked and cooled

1 Little Gem lettuce, shredded

100g (3½oz) canned black beans, drained and rinsed

1 quantity Lime & Chilli salad dressing (see page 210)

handful of coriander leaves, chopped

1 spring onion, trimmed and finely sliced

1. Preheat the oven to 200°C/180°C fan (400°F), Gas Mark 6.

2. Cover a baking tray with baking parchment and add the sweet potato cubes. Spray with low-calorie cooking spray and roast in the oven for 30 minutes, until golden brown and starting to crisp on the edges.

3. Meanwhile, cook the quinoa according to the package instructions. Set aside to cool.

4. When the sweet potato is ready, start to assemble the salad. Divide the quinoa between 2 serving bowls. Now work around the bowl (I like to do this in rainbow colour order for fun!), adding the cherry tomatoes, sweet potato, sweetcorn, lettuce and black beans.

5. Finally, drizzle the dressing over each bowl, then sprinkle with the coriander and spring onion.

OPPOSITE Mexican-style Bounty Bowl (top left), Japanese-style Bounty Bowl (middle) and English Garden Bounty Bowl (below left).

JAPANESE-STYLE BOUNTY BOWL

CALORIES PER SERVING: 267

100g (3½oz) long-grain brown rice

100g (3½oz) cucumber, finely sliced into rounds

2 small handfuls of baby spinach

1 medium carrot, peeled and ribboned (see method on page 134)

80g (2¾oz) cooked edamame beans

10 sugarsnap peas, sliced diagonally into bite-sized pieces

2 radishes, very finely sliced

1 teaspoon sesame seeds

1 quantity Miso & Ginger salad dressing (see page 210)

2 spring onions, trimmed and finely sliced

1. Cook the rice according to the package instructions. When it is cooked, drain it through a sieve and run under cold water. Allow to drain fully.
2. Divide the rice between 2 bowls. Arrange the cucumber, spinach, carrot ribbons, edamame beans, sugarsnap peas and radishes on top.
3. Dry-fry the sesame seeds for a couple of minutes in a small frying pan until starting to turn golden brown.
4. Drizzle the dressing over the bowls, then sprinkle with the toasted sesame seeds and spring onions.

NOTE Prepping the ingredients for these at the weekend makes weekday lunches much easier. Simply prepare the individual ingredients and store them in separate small, sealed containers ready to pop together in a lunchbox in the morning. If you can't get hold of some of the ingredients, just substitute something similar. I use frozen edamame beans when I can't find fresh ones.

ENGLISH GARDEN BOUNTY BOWL

CALORIES PER SERVING: 310

100g (3½oz) bulgur wheat

10 asparagus tips, trimmed

80g (2¾oz) bite-sized broccoli florets

50g (1¾oz) broad beans

large handful of watercress

1 cooked beetroot, chopped

2 tomatoes, quartered

2 radishes, finely sliced

2 teaspoons sunflower seeds

1 quantity Wholegrain Mustard salad dressing (see page 210)

handful of cress

small handful of parsley leaves, finely chopped

1. Cook the bulgur wheat according to the package instructions. Allow to cool.

2. Steam or simmer the asparagus, broccoli and broad beans for 3 minutes (if I have time, I like to peel away the tougher outer shell of the broad beans to leave just the bright green and tender middle), then rinse under cold water, drain, and set aside.

3. Divide the bulgur wheat between 2 bowls. Work around the bowl, adding watercress, beetroot, tomatoes, asparagus, broccoli, broad beans and radishes.

4. Dry-fry the sunflower seeds in a small frying pan for a couple of minutes until starting to colour.

5. Divide the dressing between the 2 bowls, then scatter over the delicate cress and the parsley, and finally sprinkle with the toasted sunflower seeds.

NOTE If you have leftover radishes, make them up into a quick pickle using the method I give for carrots on page 142.

SMOKED MACKEREL SALAD WITH GARLIC AÏOLI

Smoked mackerel makes a fantastic salad ingredient – it is great-value, full-flavoured and easy to cook. The meaty fish works perfectly with the nutty grains and vegetables here, all smothered in a creamy, garlicky aïoli.

CALORIES PER SERVING: 488

FOR THE AÏOLI
4 garlic cloves, crushed
1 egg and 1 egg white
200g (7oz) fat-free Greek yogurt
1 lemon, ½ juiced, ½ cut into wedges, to serve
salt

FOR THE SALAD
80g (2¾oz) bulgur wheat
80g (2¾oz) quinoa
4 smoked mackerel fillets
150g (5½oz) broccoli florets
250g (9oz) asparagus spears, trimmed and cut into 2cm (¾ inch) pieces
4 spring onions, trimmed and sliced
pepper

1. First prepare the aïoli. In a bowl, sprinkle a large pinch of salt over the crushed garlic, add the egg and egg white, whisk up with a fork, then beat in the yogurt. When the consistency is smooth, stir in the lemon juice.

2. Put the bulgur wheat and quinoa in a saucepan, cover with boiling water to about double the depth of the grains, and simmer gently for 10 minutes. If the grains absorb all of the water, add a little more boiling water while it is cooking. When ready, drain any excess water and set aside.

3. Preheat the grill to its highest setting. Line the grill pan with foil.

4. Lay the mackerel fillets on the grill pan and grill for 5 minutes, until warmed through and browned on top.

5. In a separate pan, simmer the broccoli for 2 minutes, then add the asparagus to the pan and simmer for a further 3 minutes. Drain the vegetables.

6. In a large serving dish, mix together the bulgur wheat and quinoa with the broccoli, asparagus and spring onions.

7. Gently prise the smoked mackerel flesh away from the skin, pull it apart into bite-sized pieces and scatter over the salad.

8. Drizzle some of the aïoli over the top and season with salt and pepper, serving the rest of the aïoli and the lemon wedges on the side.

NOTE For speed, use ready-cooked grains. Add any other vegetables you like, such as green beans, sugarsnap peas or sliced radishes. Chopped chilli on top also makes a good addition.

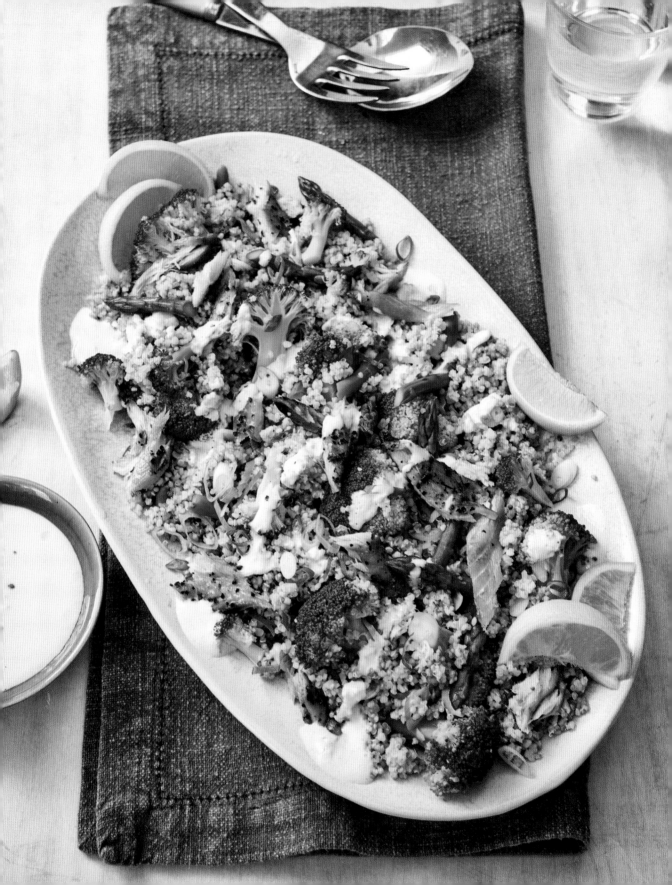

SNAPPY QUICK-PICKLED CARROTS

Tangy quick pickles are great to have in the refrigerator to add to all sorts of meals as a tasty, healthy extra on the side. Pickled carrots are delicious in salads, alongside noodle dishes or served with sandwiches. They are a fantastic way to get an extra portion of veg into your day and, as they last up to 3 weeks in the refrigerator, they're also handy for using up leftover carrots. You will need a 500ml (18fl oz) sterilized jar, with a lid that seals.

CALORIES PER SERVING: 20

300g (10½oz) carrots, peeled and cut into batons
150ml (¼ pint) white distilled vinegar
150ml (¼ pint) water
1 tablespoon honey
½ tablespoon salt

1. To sterilize your jar, preheat the oven to 180°C/160°C fan (350°F), Gas Mark 4. Wash the jar in hot, soapy water, then rinse. Place upright on a baking tray, including the lid if separate (if you are using a jar with a rubber seal, remove this before putting the jar in the oven and boil it separately for 10 minutes to sterilize). Put into the oven for 15 minutes, then allow to cool before filling.
2. Place the carrot batons into the sterilized jar.
3. In a small saucepan, mix the vinegar, measured water, honey and salt. Bring up to a rapid simmer, then stir to dissolve the salt.
4. Carefully pour the hot pickling liquid into the jar, seal it and give it a shake to make sure the carrot batons are fully submerged.
5. Allow to cool. These will be ready to serve within 2 hours or store in the refrigerator and eat within 3 weeks of opening.

NOTE Fancy some different flavours in the pickles? Try adding thyme, cumin seeds or fresh root ginger. Different ingredients will infuse their own subtle flavours into the carrots. You can also try this pickling method with radishes, cucumbers, red onions, asparagus and peppers.

BROCCOLI STEM SOUP

It's always useful to have a quick and simple soup recipe at hand when you need to whip up a quick, healthy lunch. This soup is a brilliant way to avoid wasting leftover broccoli stems, which are naturally sweet; it's tasty, wholesome and has a creamy consistency thanks to the added potato. You can take the soup up a level by stirring in some grated Cheddar or serving it with cheese on toast.

CALORIES PER SERVING: 62

low-calorie cooking spray
½ onion, finely chopped
2 garlic cloves, finely sliced
stalk and stems from
   1 head of broccoli,
   any very woody parts
   trimmed away, finely
   sliced
1 potato (about 150g / 5½oz),
   peeled and cut into cubes
700ml (1¼ pints) vegetable
   stock
½ teaspoon salt
pepper

1. Heat a saucepan with some low-calorie cooking spray and add the onion, garlic and broccoli stems. Stir-fry over a gentle heat for 6 minutes.
2. Add the potato, stock and salt, bring up to a simmer, then gently simmer for 20 minutes.
3. Using a hand blender, blend the soup until it is a smooth consistency. Serve in warmed bowls, with a little pepper ground on top.

NOTE Broccoli stems are also great sliced into coins or matchsticks and added to stir-fries, omelettes or just raw in salads. You can also roast broccoli using the same method as my Roasted Cauliflower (see page 148) to serve as a side dish.

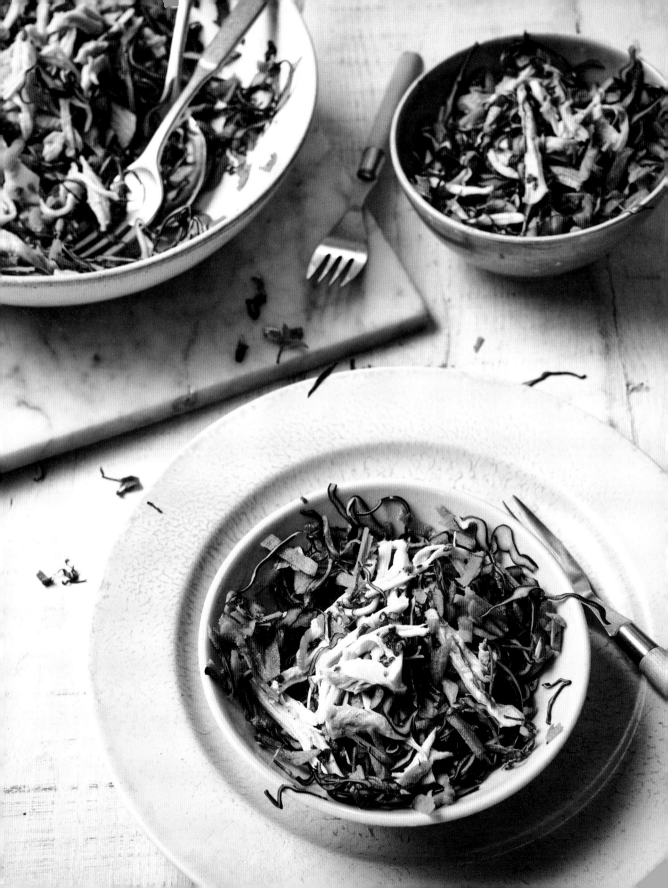

ZINGY SHREDDED THAI CHICKEN, CARROT & RED CABBAGE SALAD

This is my go-to salad for barbecues and potluck meals – it always goes down a treat and really stands out. Vibrant crisp carrot and crunchy red cabbage are tossed in a zesty, spicy dressing bursting with zing and rounded off by tasty pulled chicken.

CALORIES PER SERVING: 271

---

4 skinless chicken thigh
  fillets, excess fat trimmed
  away
low-calorie cooking spray
100ml (3½fl oz) boiling water
1 tablespoon light soy sauce
½ red cabbage, finely
  shredded
4 carrots (about 400g /
  14oz), peeled and grated
large handful of mint leaves
  (about 15g / ¼oz), roughly
  chopped

FOR THE DRESSING
1 red chilli, deseeded and
  finely chopped
2 tablespoons fish sauce
1 tablespoon honey
½ teaspoon salt
juice of 2 limes

1. First, prepare the shredded chicken. In a saucepan with a lid, fry the thigh fillets in low-calorie cooking spray for 2 minutes on each side, then cover with the measured boiling water and the soy sauce, put the lid on and simmer gently for 10 minutes.

2. Remove the chicken from the pan and shred straightaway, using 2 forks to pull it apart. Set the chicken aside while you assemble the salad.

3. Put the cabbage, carrots and mint in a large bowl, then place the shredded chicken on top.

4. Mix all the dressing ingredients together in a small bowl. Pour the dressing over the salad and toss to combine with your hands or some salad servers.

NOTE This recipe is a great way to use up leftover roast chicken. You could also replace the chicken with grilled halloumi, if you prefer. If you have a food processor with a grating attachment, this salad is even easier to make, as you can prepare the carrot and red cabbage very quickly.

CHILLI ROASTED VEGETABLES

Roasting vegetables both tenderizes them and brings out incredible flavours. These are sweet, caramelized and have a kick of chilli, making a fantastic side to many dishes – try them with quiches, roast meats or pasta – or a tasty base for a soup. Sometimes I like to make up a batch of these at the weekend, so I have an extra portion of vegetables in the refrigerator to add to my meals during the week.

CALORIES PER SERVING: 131

2 small/medium aubergines, roughly chopped

250g (9oz) cherry tomatoes, halved

2 courgettes, cut into chunks

2 peppers (red, orange or yellow), deseeded and chopped

2 medium sweet potatoes, peeled and chopped

2 red onions, sliced

1 tablespoon Italian seasoning

2 teaspoons chilli flakes

4 tablespoons balsamic vinegar

low-calorie cooking spray

salt and pepper

1. Preheat the oven to 220°C/200°C fan (425°F), Gas Mark 7.
2. Throw all the vegetables into an extra-large roasting tin with the Italian seasoning, chilli flakes and balsamic vinegar, then season with salt and pepper and give everything a good mix. Spray generously with low-calorie cooking spray and mix again.
3. Put the vegetables into the oven and roast for 25 minutes, then give everything another good stir and roast for another 20 minutes.
4. The vegetables should be soft and starting to brown and caramelize a little. If they are still looking a little underdone, give them another stir and pop them back into the oven. Check at 10-minute intervals until they are done.

NOTE Roasted vegetables are a great way to use up leftovers that might otherwise be thrown away. Try adding mushrooms, butternut squash, garlic, celery, broccoli, green beans, parsnips, carrots, asparagus or even Brussels sprouts.

CANNELLINI BEAN MASH

For when you just don't have time to make mashed potatoes. This mash can be ready from start to finish in 5 minutes and pairs perfectly with stews and casseroles, or even sausages and gravy. Try it alongside Easy Spanish Chicken & Chorizo Stew, Cowgirls' Stew, Italian Chicken Cacciatore or Pot-roast Beef Brisket with Hasselback Carrots (see pages 64, 70, 84 and 122).

**CALORIES PER
SERVING: 145**

low-calorie cooking spray
1 garlic clove, crushed
2 × 400g (14oz) cans
   cannellini beans,
   drained and rinsed
100ml (3½fl oz) vegetable
   stock
salt and pepper

1. Spray a small saucepan with low-calorie cooking spray, add the garlic, bring it up to a sizzle and cook for just 30 seconds, long enough for the fragrance to come out, but being careful not to burn it. Add the cannellini beans and stock to the pan, bring up to a simmer and cook for 5 minutes.
2. Remove from the heat and mash with a potato masher until smooth. The mash may appear quite liquidy at first, but as you crush the beans they will absorb the moisture.
3. Season to taste with salt and pepper and serve.

NOTE You can add herbs such as rosemary and thyme to this, to complement the dish you are serving it with, or even try finely grated lemon zest. You can also replace the cannellini beans with butter beans.

ROASTED CAULIFLOWER

This is by far my favourite way to eat cauliflower. Roasting brings out its nutty and buttery taste, and gives little crispy edges that add texture and make it irresistible. This is lovely just with a little salt, but you can also jazz it up with spice mixes (see pages 212–13) to go with whatever you are eating: peri-peri is my favourite.

CALORIES PER SERVING: 46

1 cauliflower, leaves and stalk removed, cut into bite-sized florets
low-calorie cooking spray
salt, or spice mix of your choice (see recipe introduction)

1. Preheat the oven to 240°C/220°C fan (475°F), Gas Mark 9.
2. Cover a baking tray with baking parchment, spread the cauliflower over it in an even layer and spray with low-calorie cooking spray.
3. Grind some salt over the top or add 1 tablespoon of the spice mix of your choice.
4. Roast for 15 minutes, then remove from the oven and use a spatula to flip the cauliflower over, before roasting for another 10 minutes. The cauliflower will be golden in places, with a few little blackened edges.

NOTE Cauliflower 'rice' is also easy to make and can be a great light side dish to replace white rice. Simply remove the leaves from a cauliflower, quarter it and remove the core, then chop each quarter into 3 pieces. Pulse the cauliflower in a food processor until it is finely chopped. Spread the 'rice' out on a baking tray, spray with low-calorie cooking spray and roast for 10 minutes in an oven preheated to 220°C/200°C fan (425°F), Gas Mark 7.

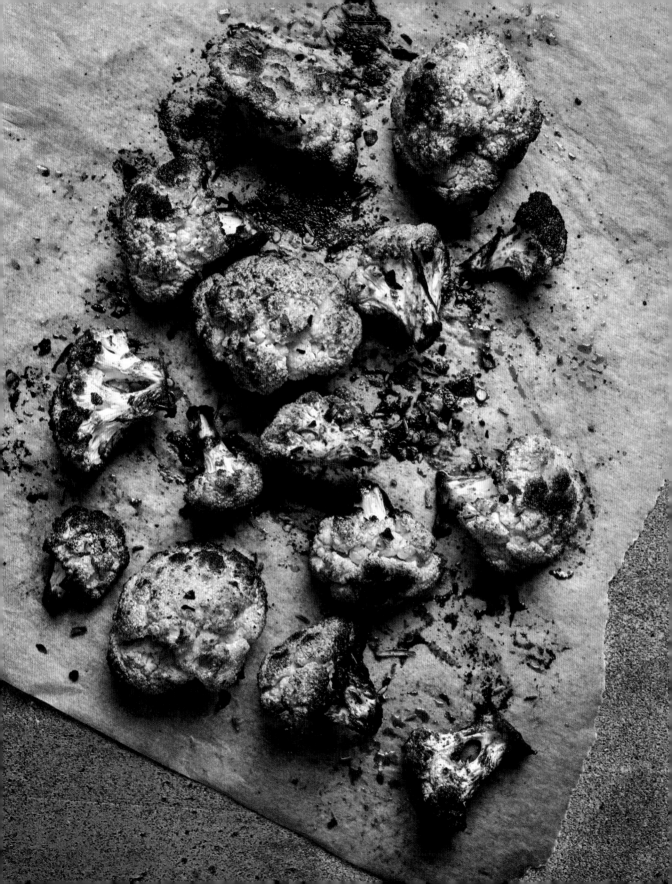

BAKED SWEET POTATO WEDGES

Sweet potato wedges make a brilliant side to so many different meals and the crisp edges are irresistible with that soft, caramelized inside. You can season these however you like so that they fit perfectly with your meal – try 1 tablespoon of any of the spice mixes on pages 212–13 mixed into the wedges before they are baked. Garlic Aïoli (see page 140) makes a delicious dip for these.

CALORIES PER SERVING: 170

4 large sweet potatoes
   (about 750g / 1lb 10oz),
   peeled
low-calorie cooking spray
salt, or spice mix of your
   choice (see recipe
   introduction)

1. Preheat the oven to 220°C/200°C fan (425°F), Gas Mark 7.
2. Make the wedges by cutting each potato in half lengthways, then cut each half into 4 or 6 pieces, depending on the size of the potato.
3. Line a large baking tray with foil and spray with low-calorie cooking spray.
4. If using one of the spice mixes from pages 212–13, place the wedges in a large bowl, spray with cooking spray and add 1 tablespoon of the spice mix, then stir to coat evenly.
5. Place the wedges, peeled side down, on the baking tray, spread out evenly, and spray them generously with cooking spray.
6. Place them in the oven and bake for 30 minutes, turning halfway through.
7. When they are done, they will be golden on the outside, perhaps with some slightly blackened edges, and the insides will be soft.
8. Season with salt once they are cooked and serve immediately.

NOTE To make tasty wedges with regular white potatoes, follow the same method, but add 5–10 minutes onto the cooking time to get them crispy on the outside and soft in the middle.

SERVES 4

PERFECT OVEN-BAKED CHIPS

This is how I make hot, crispy, seasoned oven-baked chips that are a great treat alongside dishes such as The Classic Sloppy Joe, Crunchy Pea & Mint Fish Bites or Peri-peri Chicken with Sweetcorn Salsa (see pages 95, 104 and 165).

CALORIES PER SERVING: 178

1kg (2lb 4oz) floury
  potatoes, such as Maris
  Piper, peeled
low-calorie cooking spray
freshly ground salt

1. Preheat the oven to 220°C/200°C fan (425°F), Gas Mark 7.
2. Cut the peeled potatoes into thick batons, placing them into a large saucepan of cold water as you cut them.
3. Place a lid on the pan over a high heat and bring the water to the boil, then reduce the heat to medium and simmer for 3 minutes. Drain, then leave the chips steaming in the colander for a few minutes to dry out.
4. Cover an extra-large baking tray, or 2 smaller trays, with baking parchment, spray it with low-calorie cooking spray, place the chips on the tray – spacing them out as much as possible – and spray generously with more cooking spray.
5. Grind some salt over the chips, then place them on the top shelf of the oven for 20 minutes.
6. Remove them from the oven, use a spatula to flip them over, spray again with cooking spray and bake for another 20 minutes. They should be golden and crisp on the outside and fluffy on the inside.

NOTE You can season these to make them more interesting or to match whatever you are cooking. Try any of the spice mixes on pages 212–13 – simply mix in 1–2 tablespoons of the spice mix before spraying with cooking spray.

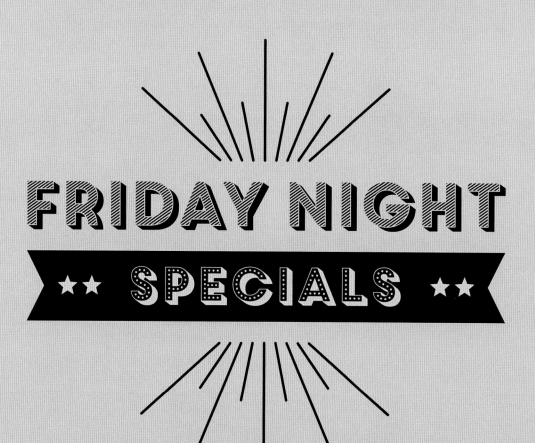

• • • • • • • • • • • • •

I love to plan slightly more indulgent meals for the weekend and I especially look forward to a treat on a Friday night. It's so easy to prepare a takeaway-style option at home for a fraction of the calories in a ready meal or 'proper' takeaway, and it's so much more budget-friendly to make your own.

I cannot resist a good chicken tikka masala – and the slow cooker Tick-tock Tikka Masala version in this chapter is creamy enough to feel like a real splurge – plus you can put it in the slow cooker in the morning so you don't have to do any hard work later on. I love a curry feast at the weekend and often cook up a vegetarian curry (which also gives leftovers for the week ahead) or a couple of quick side dishes to go alongside. My 5-minute Saag Dhal and Jeera Aloo are ideal for this: both are quick to make and add an extra dimension to the main curry.

If you're feeling a bit more adventurous, Prawn Noodles with *Nam Jim* Sauce is another real favourite of mine. The depth of flavour that comes from this combination of ingredients is unique, but still easy to cook at home. Returning to more familiar flavours, a Mexican-style feast is another of my weekend heroes. Try Slow-cooker Mexican Beef with Lime & Coriander Rice (see page 154) and some Zucchimole (see page 208): so tasty.

For weekends when we have visitors, I like to make some meals ahead so I don't spend the whole time cooking. The Weekend Veggie Chilli is perfect for this, and again can be dressed up with some easy side dishes, or a big platter of Crunchy Tandoori Chicken with Homemade Minty Coleslaw is a great meal to share.

• • • • • • • • • • • • •

SERVES 4
SPICY PEANUT AUBERGINE CURRY
WITH LIME & CORIANDER RICE

Aubergines have a robust texture and are great meat substitutes – here they soak up the flavours of this sauce and almost melt into it.

CALORIES PER SERVING: 451

FOR THE CURRY
2 aubergines (about 700g / 1lb 9oz total weight), chopped into small chunks

2 red peppers, deseeded and chopped

low-calorie cooking spray

2 tablespoons smooth peanut butter

3 tablespoons dark soy sauce

1 tablespoon rice vinegar

1 red chilli

2 garlic cloves, peeled

1 tablespoon sweet chilli sauce

300ml (½ pint boiling water)

35g (1¼oz) unsalted peanuts, crushed, to serve

FOR THE RICE
300g (10½oz) white basmati rice

finely grated zest and juice of 1 unwaxed lime

finely chopped coriander

1. In a sauté pan, fry the aubergines and peppers in low-calorie cooking spray over a gentle heat for 15 minutes, stirring occasionally.

2. Make up the sauce in a mini chopper. Spoon the peanut butter into the bowl with the soy sauce, rice vinegar, red chilli, garlic and sweet chilli sauce and blend until smooth.

3. Once the aubergine and pepper have been frying for 15 minutes, add the sauce, stir well, then top up with the measured boiling water. Simmer for 30 minutes, stirring occasionally and topping up with a splash more boiling water if it starts to look too dry.

4. Halfway through the curry cooking time, put the basmati rice on to cook, according to the package instructions.

5. When the rice is cooked and fluffy, drain, then stir in the lime zest and juice and the chopped coriander.

6. Crush the peanuts in a pestle and mortar, or put the peanuts in a sandwich bag and bash them with a rolling pin. When they're crushed, place them in a small, dry frying pan and set over a high heat, stir-frying for a couple of minutes until golden brown and smelling delicious.

7. Serve up the rice, spoon the curry over the top and scatter with the toasted peanuts.

NOTE Try swapping the white rice for brown basmati rice for a slightly more chewy consistency (you will need to cook it for longer, so follow the package instructions).

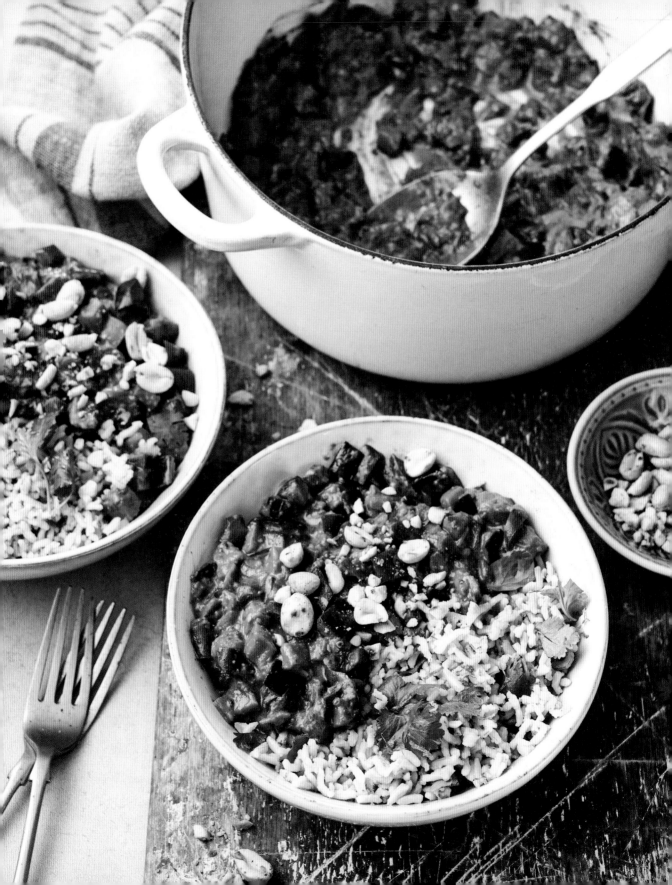

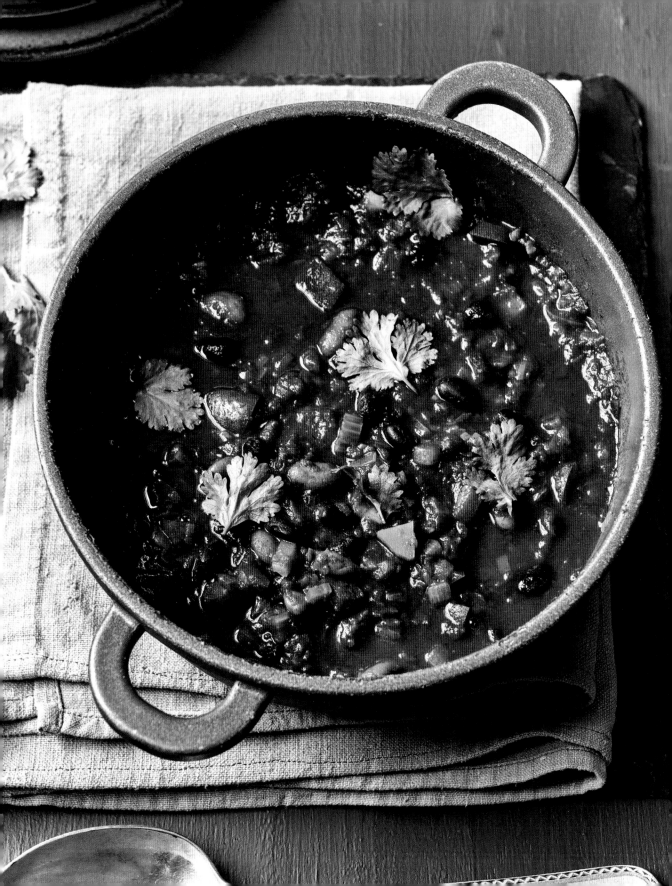

WEEKEND VEGGIE CHILLI

A warming bowl of this hearty chilli can't be beaten with its spicy, smoky and sweet flavours. Serve it with melting cheese and alongside some Zucchimole (see page 208) to take it to the next level for your guests.

**CALORIES PER
SERVING: 282**

1 large onion, finely chopped

2 celery sticks, finely chopped

1 leek, finely chopped

low-calorie cooking spray

4 garlic cloves, crushed

2 large carrots, peeled and
   finely chopped

3 red peppers, deseeded and
   chopped

2 × 400g (14oz) cans
   chopped tomatoes

350ml (12fl oz) water

400g (14oz) can black beans,
   drained and rinsed

400g (14oz) can pinto beans,
   drained and rinsed

3 tablespoons tomato purée

2 tablespoons dark soy sauce

1 tablespoon red wine vinegar

handful of coriander, to serve

FOR THE SPICE MIX

2 teaspoons chilli powder

2 teaspoons ground cumin

2 teaspoons smoked paprika

1 teaspoon salt

1. Preheat the oven to 200°C/180°C fan (400°F), Gas Mark 6.

2. Mix all the spices for the spice mix together in a small bowl.

3. In a large ovenproof casserole dish, fry the onion, celery and leek in low-calorie cooking spray for 10 minutes, then add the garlic, carrots and peppers. Stir-fry for 2 minutes.

4. Pour in the tomatoes, water, black beans and pinto beans, then add the tomato purée, soy sauce, vinegar and spice mix and stir everything together thoroughly.

5. Bring up to a rapid simmer, then put a lid on and place in the oven to cook for 1 hour. When ready, the chilli should be a rich dark colour and all the vegetables tender.

6. Serve scattered with coriander.

NOTE This is a great way to use up leftover vegetables. Sweet potato, butternut squash, parsnips, mushrooms or sweetcorn kernels all make great additions. This can be made in advance and just reheated when needed, and any leftovers can be frozen.

GOLDEN COCONUT CURRY WITH BUTTERNUT SQUASH & RED LENTILS

Serve this creamy, subtly sweet and spicy curry with rice or Quick & Easy Wholemeal 3-ingredient Flatbreads (see page 188) and fat-free Greek yogurt.

CALORIES PER SERVING: 203

1 onion, finely chopped

3 garlic cloves, crushed

5cm (2 inch) piece of fresh root ginger, peeled and grated

1 red chilli, deseeded and finely chopped

500g (1lb 2oz) butternut squash, chopped into 1cm (½ inch) cubes

120g (4¼oz) red lentils

450ml (16fl oz) vegetable stock

400g (14oz) can chopped tomatoes

400g (14oz) can light coconut milk

2 teaspoons ground turmeric

½ teaspoon mustard seeds

1 teaspoon cumin seeds

1 teaspoon garam masala

1 teaspoon salt

50g (1¾oz) spinach

1. Preheat the oven to 180°C/160°C fan (350°F), Gas Mark 4.
2. Put all the ingredients except the spinach in a large casserole dish with a lid, give everything a good stir, then place the lid on.
3. Cook in the oven for 1½ hours, stirring halfway through.
4. When the curry comes out of the oven, stir in the spinach and serve.

NOTE To make this in a slow cooker, cook for 4 hours on high, or 8 hours on low.

ONE OF THE EASIEST WAYS TO REMOVE THE SKIN FROM A BUTTERNUT SQUASH IS TO USE A Y-SHAPED POTATO PEELER. YOU CAN ALSO USE FROZEN PRE-PREPARED BUTTERNUT SQUASH, IF YOU PREFER.

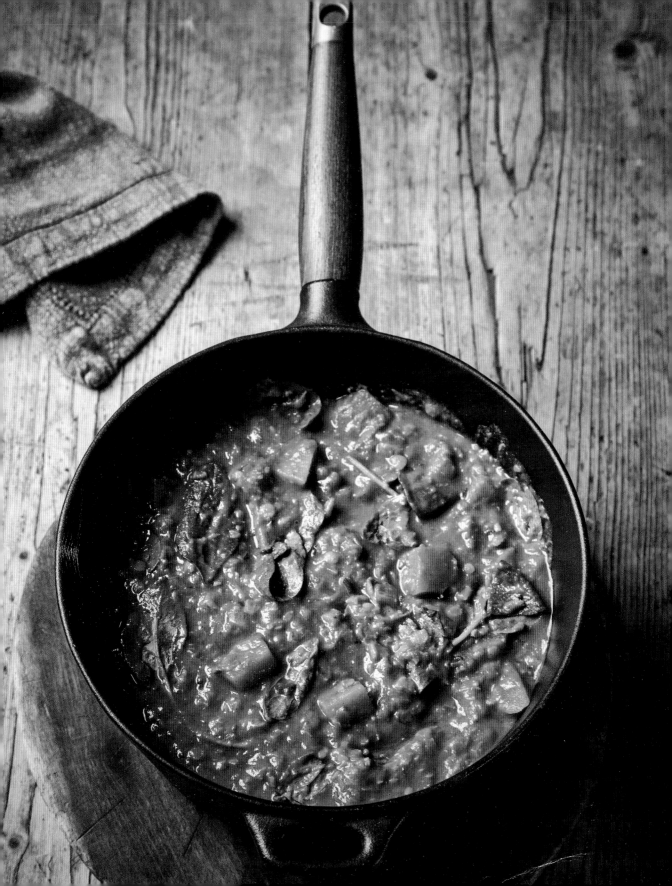

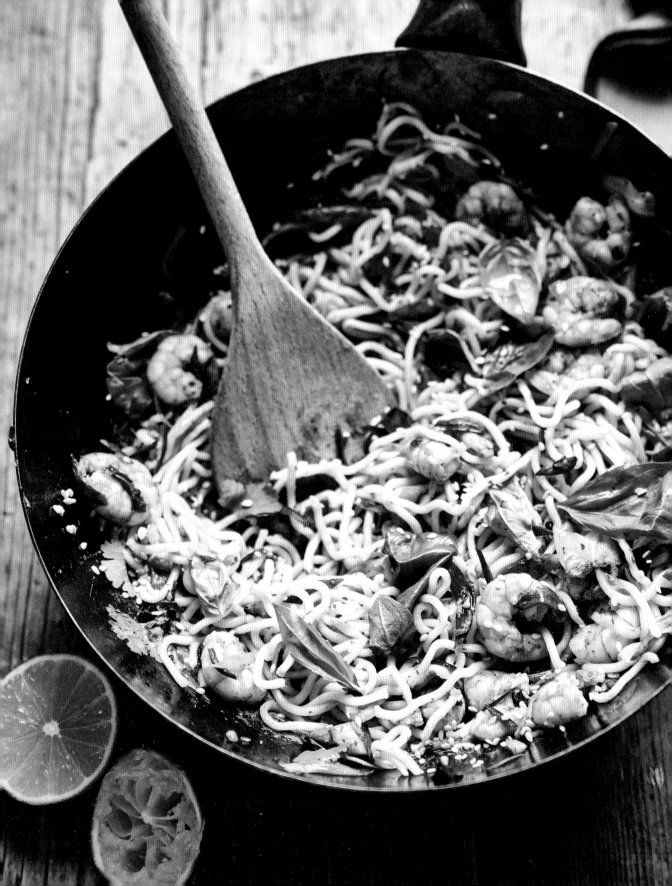

PRAWN NOODLES WITH NAM JIM SAUCE

Mouth-wateringly tangy noodles with prawns, chilli and lime, these simply explode with flavour and are one of my favourite Friday night treats. Using ready-cooked noodles makes it extra quick to prepare.

CALORIES PER SERVING: 379

160g (5¾oz) raw king prawns

2 garlic cloves, crushed

½ teaspoon olive oil

1 shallot, finely chopped

2 tablespoons fish sauce

2 teaspoons tamarind paste

1 teaspoon ancho chilli flakes (or see note, below)

1 tablespoon maple syrup

large handful of coriander (about 20g / ¾oz), finely chopped

juice of 1 lime, plus extra lime wedges, to serve

300g (10½oz) pre-cooked medium noodles

3 spring onions, trimmed and cut on the diagonal into 5mm (¼ inch) slices

2 red chillies, deseeded and finely chopped

small handful of basil leaves

½ teaspoon sesame seeds

salt

1. In a small bowl, mix the prawns with the crushed garlic, a pinch of salt and the olive oil. Set aside while prepping the other ingredients.
2. To make the sauce, mix together the shallot, fish sauce, tamarind paste, ancho chilli flakes, maple syrup, half the chopped coriander and the lime juice.
3. Make sure all the other ingredients are chopped and ready, as you'll need to move quickly now!
4. Set a sauté pan or wok over a medium-high heat and add the prawns. Stir-fry for 1½ minutes, until the prawns are pink.
5. Loosen the noodles up a bit and add them to the pan, then add the sauce. Give everything a good stir, coating the noodles in the sauce.
6. Add the spring onions, chillies, basil and the remaining coriander and stir-fry everything together for about 1 minute.
7. Scatter the sesame seeds over the top, and serve with lime wedges on the side.

NOTE If you find it hard to get hold of ancho chilli flakes, then another smoky chilli will do in their place, such as chipotle.

CRUNCHY TANDOORI CHICKEN

WITH HOMEMADE MINTY COLESLAW

Succulent spiced chicken and a crisp, minty coleslaw: a perfect pairing.

CALORIES PER SERVING: 569

2 tablespoons tandoori curry powder

150g (5½oz) fat-free Greek yogurt

8 skinless chicken thigh fillets, excess fat trimmed away

75g (2¾oz) cornflakes

low-calorie cooking spray

salt

FOR THE COLESLAW

½ red cabbage, finely shredded

2 carrots, peeled and julienned, or coarsely grated

3 spring onions, trimmed and cut on the diagonal into 1cm (½ inch) slices

juice of 1 lemon

handful of mint leaves (about 15g / ½oz), shredded

salt and pepper

1. In a large bowl, stir the curry powder and a pinch of salt into the yogurt, then add the chicken and coat it all over in the spiced yogurt. Cover the bowl and allow to marinate for at least 30 minutes.

2. Preheat the oven to 220°C/200°C fan (425°F), Gas Mark 7.

3. Crush the cornflakes into fine crumbs, either in a food processor or by placing them in a food bag and crushing with a rolling pin or your hands.

4. Spray a baking tray with low-calorie cooking spray (line it with foil if using a nonstick tray).

5. When the chicken has marinated, remove each piece, shake off any excess yogurt, then dip it in the crushed cornflakes until well coated.

6. Place the coated chicken on the baking tray, spray generously with cooking spray and put into the oven for 25 minutes (have a peek at 20 minutes, just to check that they aren't starting to burn).

7. Meanwhile, make the coleslaw. Simply toss all the ingredients together in a large bowl and season to taste with salt and pepper.

8. When the chicken is ready, the outside will be golden brown and crisp, and the inside cooked through and perfectly tender. (Pierce one of the largest pieces: if the juices run clear with no traces of pink, it is ready.) Serve with the coleslaw.

NOTE Coating a whole chicken in the same marinade before roasting puts a new twist on a roast dinner.

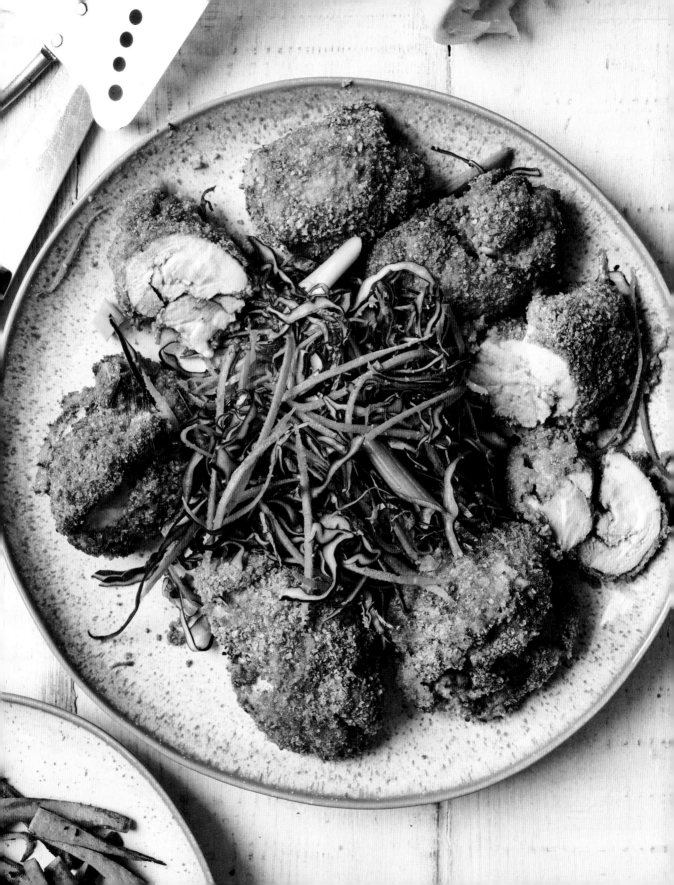

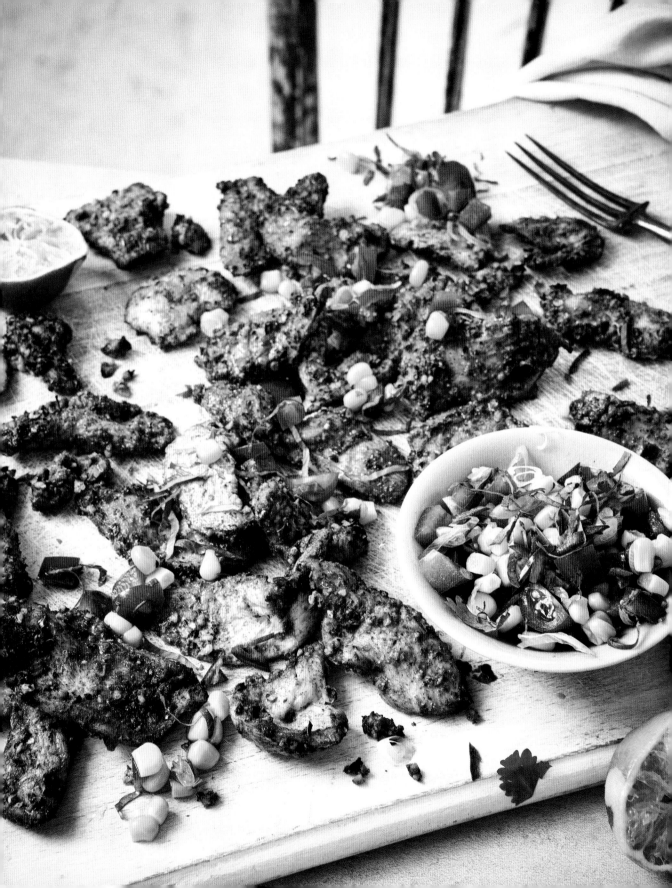

PERI-PERI CHICKEN
WITH SWEETCORN SALSA

Fiery peri-peri chicken is a winner served with crunchy, zingy sweetcorn salsa. Marinating the chicken leaves it tender, even after grilling. Serve with homemade Perfect Oven-baked Chips (see page 151) or rice.

**CALORIES PER
SERVING: 278**

2 tablespoons Peri-peri
  spice mix (see page 212)
4 chicken breasts, cut into
  strips
100ml (3½fl oz) semi-
  skimmed milk

FOR THE SALSA
160g (5¾oz) frozen
  sweetcorn, cooked and
  cooled
2 spring onions, trimmed
  and finely sliced
12 cherry tomatoes, finely
  chopped
1 red pepper, deseeded and
  finely chopped
1 red chilli, finely chopped
small handful of coriander
  leaves and stalks, finely
  chopped
juice of 1 lime
salt

1. In a small bowl, mix the peri-peri spices with the chicken strips until coated, then pour over the milk. Mix again, then cover and marinate for at least 1 hour.
2. Preheat the grill on its highest setting. Once the chicken has marinated, lay the strips out on a grill pan, and grill on high for 4–5 minutes on each side.
3. Meanwhile, make up the sweetcorn salsa. Put the sweetcorn in a bowl and add the spring onions, tomatoes, red pepper, chilli and coriander. Add a pinch of salt, then pour over the lime juice. Stir everything together to combine thoroughly.
4. When the chicken strips are ready, they should be golden brown on the outside, with no pink remaining in the middle. Serve them with the salsa.

NOTE This meal is perfect for a barbecue. You can prepare the chicken the day before and marinate it overnight, covered, in the refrigerator. It's also easy to make up extra chicken to keep in the refrigerator for tasty lunchtime wraps or to add to salads.

TICK-TOCK TIKKA MASALA

I don't think you can beat a steaming bowl of creamy, fragrant chicken tikka masala, and being able to just put it in the slow cooker and leave it to do its thing is so satisfying. Takeaway and ready-meal versions of this are usually packed with calories, but this is just as delicious (if not more so). Serve with basmati rice and, if you fancy a little bit of a curry feast, why not try adding a couple of easy sides, such as Jeera Aloo or 5-minute Saag Dhal (see pages 172 and 174.)

CALORIES PER SERVING: 291

1 tablespoon peeled and finely chopped fresh root ginger

3 garlic cloves, crushed

1 tablespoon ground cumin

1 tablespoon garam masala

1 teaspoon ground turmeric

1 teaspoon ground coriander

3 cardamom pods

½ tablespoon chilli powder

1 teaspoon salt

4 chicken breasts, chopped into chunks

250ml (9fl oz) tomato passata

200g (7oz) light coconut milk

100g (3½oz) fat-free Greek yogurt

1 tablespoon cornflour

nigella seeds, to serve

1. Put the ginger, garlic, spices, salt, chicken, passata and coconut milk into the slow cooker bowl.

2. Cook on high for 4 hours, or on low for 8 hours. When cooked, uncover and allow to cool for 10 minutes.

3. Mix the yogurt and cornflour together in a small bowl. Leave for 5 minutes.

4. Spoon the yogurt mixture on top of the curry and leave it a couple of minutes to warm through (this brings up the temperature of the yogurt, to prevent curdling). Now stir the yogurt mixture into the curry, replace the lid and leave for 15 minutes to thicken.

5. Taste and adjust the seasoning if needed. Remove the cardamom pods, if you can find them (or warn your guests to do so), and serve sprinkled with nigella seeds.

NOTE Want to make this in the oven instead? Simply start by frying the chicken in low-calorie cooking spray in a casserole dish for about 5 minutes. Add the ginger and garlic and stir-fry for another 2 minutes. Stir through the spices and salt for about a minute, then add the passata and coconut milk. Put into an oven preheated to 180°C/160°C fan (350°F), Gas Mark 4, for 1 hour. Remove from the oven, spoon on the yogurt and cornflour mixture, give it a couple of minutes to warm through a bit, then stir through before serving.

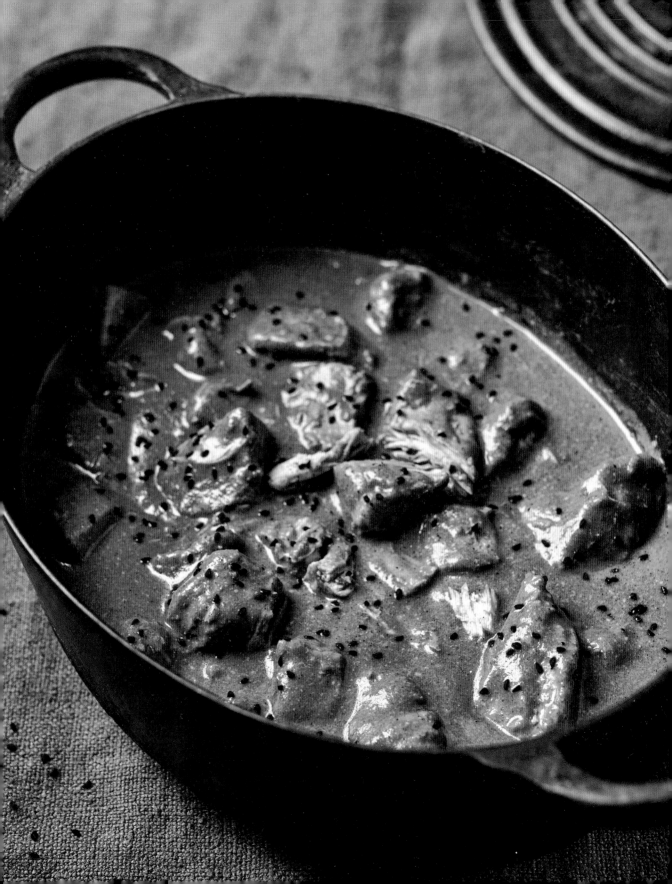

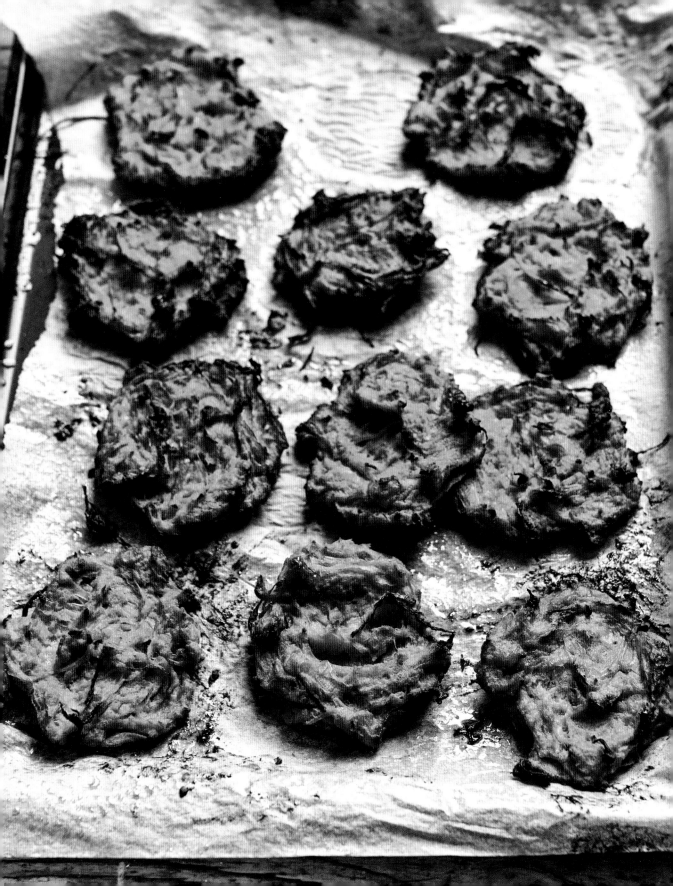

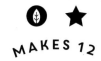

SWEET POTATO BAKED ONION BHAJIS

Soft, sweet onions are encased in a light, Indian-inspired, spiced sweet potato batter, then baked in the oven to reduce the amount of oil that would be needed if you were deep-frying them. The oven baking also gives them a very satisfying crunch on the outside. Serve these alongside a curry or dhal, or simply have them as a delicious healthy snack.

CALORIES PER BHAJI: 42

4 onions, finely sliced
low-calorie cooking spray
2 small sweet potatoes,
   pricked and microwaved
   for 7 minutes
1 egg
½ teaspoon ground turmeric
½ teaspoon ground cumin
½ teaspoon chilli powder
½ teaspoon salt

1. Preheat the oven to 200°C/180°C fan (400°F), Gas Mark 6.
2. Fry the onions gently in low-calorie cooking spray for about 10 minutes, until soft and golden. Remove from the heat and allow to cool for a few minutes.
3. Scoop the flesh out of the cooked sweet potatoes into a bowl and mash with a fork.
4. Add the egg, spices and salt to the sweet potato, using the fork to combine thoroughly to make a batter. Stir in the cooled fried onions until thoroughly coated.
5. Line a baking tray with baking parchment and use your hands to shape bhajis out of the mixture (this should make about 12).
6. Spray thoroughly with cooking spray and bake for 45 minutes until golden and crisp.

NOTE Try making a quick yogurt and mint dip to go with these. Simply mix 250g (9oz) fat-free Greek yogurt, a handful of finely chopped mint leaves, 1 crushed garlic clove, 1 tablespoon lemon juice and a pinch of salt in a small bowl.

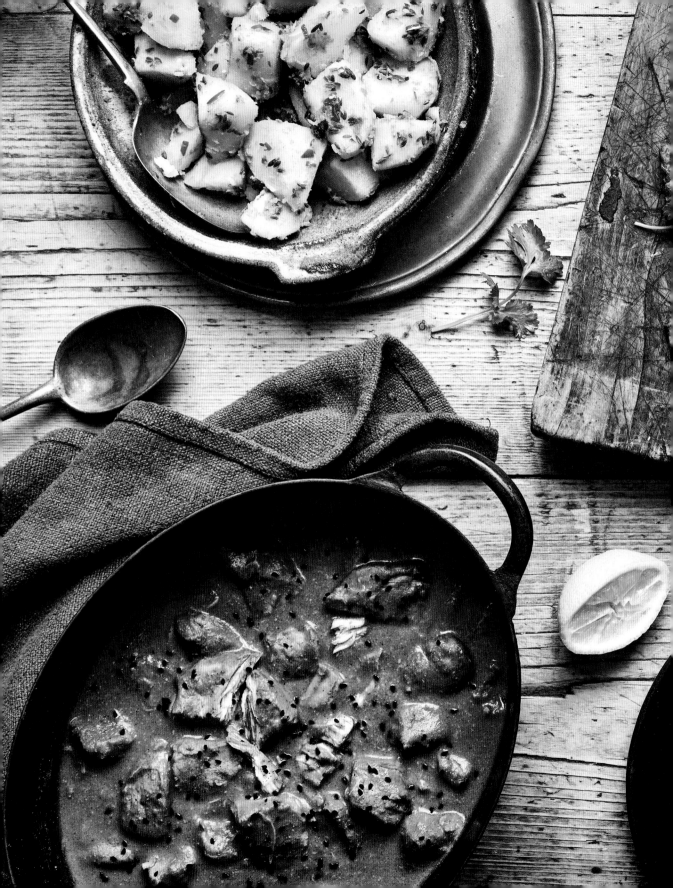

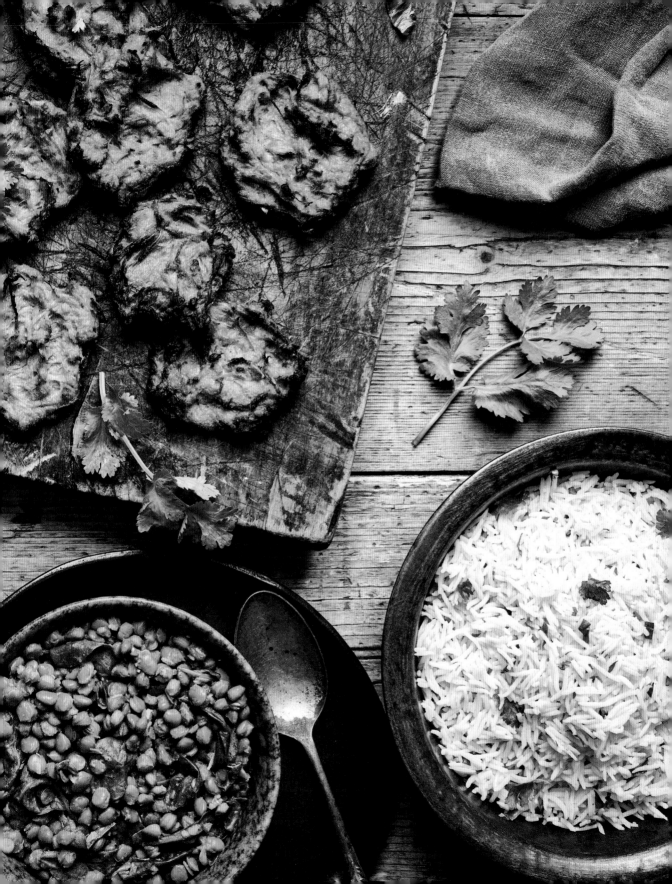

JEERA ALOO

This was one of the first Indian dishes I ever tried as a child and I was instantly in love! The potatoes are gently spiced with cumin and make a perfect quick and filling side dish. With this version I have included some chilli, but it can easily be omitted for those times when you need a side dish for chilli-shy friends.

CALORIES PER SERVING: 145

750g (1lb 10oz) potatoes, peeled and cut into chunks
2 teaspoons cumin seeds
2 green chillies, deseeded and finely chopped
5cm (2 inch) piece of fresh root ginger, peeled and grated
½ teaspoon ground turmeric
4 tablespoons water
½ teaspoon salt
juice of 1 lemon

1. Cook the potato chunks for 15 minutes in a saucepan of boiling water, until cooked through, then drain and set aside to steam.
2. Set a dry frying pan over a medium heat, add the cumin seeds, green chillies, ginger and turmeric and stir-fry for 1 minute. Add the measured water, mix it into the spices, then add the potatoes. Add the salt and lemon juice and stir-fry for 2–3 minutes.
3. Serve immediately.

NOTE If you'd like a slightly lighter option, you can always replace the potato with cauliflower. Just simmer the cauliflower for 5 minutes initially, rinse with cold water, then set aside to add into the sauce once the chilli and spices have been fried.

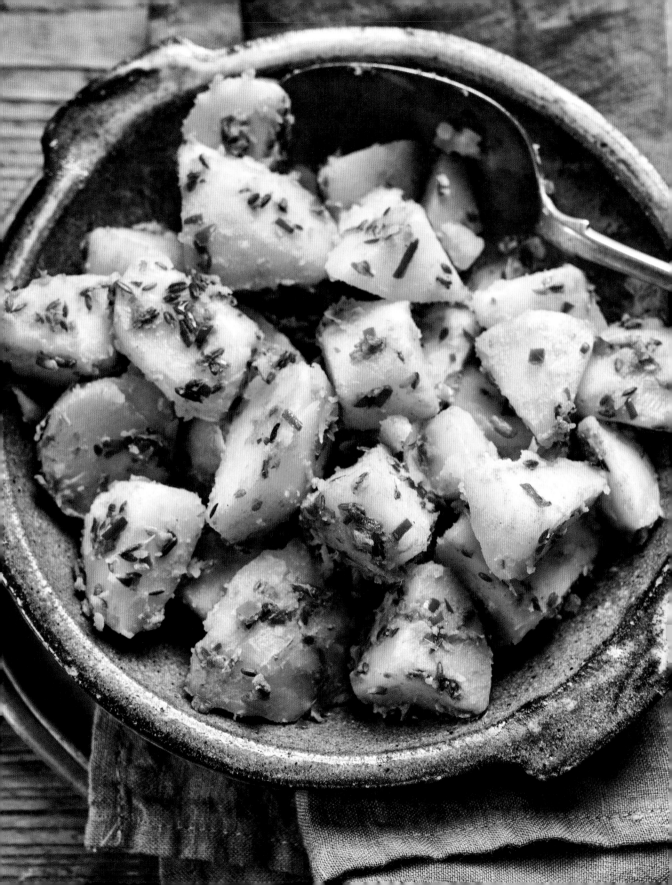

5-MINUTE SAAG DHAL

A lightning-quick side dish that makes an ideal accompaniment to any curry, with fragrant spinach and earthy lentils dressed with zesty lemon juice. See photograph on page 170–1.

CALORIES PER SERVING: 111

low-calorie cooking spray
1 garlic clove, crushed
1 green chilli, finely chopped
1 teaspoon cumin seeds
1 teaspoon ground turmeric
1 teaspoon garam masala
½ teaspoon salt
400g (14oz) can green lentils, drained and rinsed
2 tablespoons water
300g (10½oz) baby spinach, roughly chopped
juice of 1 lemon

1. Spray a sauté pan with a lid with low-calorie cooking spray and set it over a high heat. Add the garlic, chilli, cumin seeds, turmeric, garam masala and salt, and stir-fry quickly for 30 seconds.
2. Tip in the lentils and stir-fry for another 30 seconds, then spoon in the measured water.
3. Keeping the heat on high, add the spinach to the pan and stir-fry for 1 minute. Cover the pan, reduce the heat slightly and allow to cook for 3 minutes.
4. The spinach should now be wilted. Give everything a thorough stir, remove from the heat and dress with the lemon juice before serving.

NOTE Want to make this quick side dish even more super-speedy? Swap in garlic paste from a jar, pre-chopped chilli and frozen spinach!

RICH LAMB CURRY

When possible, and if I have the time, I like to prepare two curries for one meal as a weekend treat. Typically one will be sweeter and creamier with a lighter sauce, but the other needs to be dark with rich flavours. I find that lamb can be quite a fragrant meat, but in this curry it balances well with a mix of earthy spices and sweet onion to create that contrasting curry I'm looking for. It's also beautiful simply served with basmati rice.

CALORIES PER SERVING: 396

5 tablespoons fat-free Greek yogurt
1 teaspoon ground turmeric
1 teaspoon chilli powder
500g (1lb 2oz) lamb neck fillet, or lamb leg steaks, chopped into even-sized chunks
4 red onions, finely chopped
2 teaspoons cumin seeds
low-calorie cooking spray
1 tablespoon peeled and finely grated fresh root ginger
4 garlic cloves, crushed
2 green chillies, finely chopped
1 teaspoon ground cumin
1 teaspoon ground coriander
1 teaspoon garam masala
1 teaspoon salt
600ml (20fl oz) hot water
4 tablespoons tomato purée
a few mint leaves, chopped, to serve

1. Mix together the yogurt, turmeric and chilli powder in a bowl, then add the lamb and stir. Cover and set aside while you make the sauce.

2. Stir-fry the onions and cumin seeds in low-calorie cooking spray for 8 minutes, until the onions are browned and caramelizing. Add the ginger, garlic and green chillies and stir-fry for a minute. Add the ground spices and salt and stir through the onion mix. Pour in 100ml (3½fl oz) of the hot water, add the tomato purée and stir everything together.

3. Add the lamb and yogurt mixture to the pan and fry for 7 minutes, stirring regularly. Pour in the remaining hot water, stir well, then allow to simmer for 40 minutes, stirring occasionally.

4. When ready to serve, the sauce will be thick and rich, and the lamb tender.

5. Sprinkle with the chopped mint to serve.

NOTE This is a great dish for using up leftover roast lamb – simply mix it into the yogurt mixture after it has been simmering for 20 minutes, so it simmers for the final 20 minutes.

SINGAPORE NOODLES

These were always a takeaway favourite of mine, fine noodles flavoured and richly yellow-coloured with curry powder, packed with pork, prawns and crunchy vegetables. You can use rice vermicelli noodles, but I don't always find them easy to get hold of, so I make this with fine egg noodles, which work just as well.

CALORIES PER SERVING: 437

2 nests (125g / 4½oz) fine egg noodles

2 pork loin steaks (about 250g / 9oz total weight), fat trimmed away, finely sliced

1 teaspoon Chinese 5 spice powder

1 tablespoon soy sauce

1 tablespoon rice wine

2 teaspoons curry powder

½ teaspoon ground turmeric

½ teaspoon honey

low-calorie cooking spray

80g (2¾oz) frozen cold-water prawns, defrosted

2 garlic cloves, crushed

3 spring onions, trimmed and finely sliced

½ red pepper, deseeded and finely sliced

60g (2¼oz) mangetout

1 red chilli, deseeded and finely sliced, to serve

1. Cook the noodles according to the package instructions, then drain, run under cold water and set aside.
2. Mix the sliced pork with the Chinese 5 spice powder.
3. Mix the soy sauce, rice wine, curry powder, turmeric and honey together in a small bowl to make up the sauce.
4. Set a wok or sauté pan over a high heat and fry the pork in low-calorie cooking spray for 2 minutes. Add the prawns and stir-fry for 30 seconds.
5. Add the garlic, spring onions, red pepper and mangetout and stir-fry for 1½ minutes.
6. Stir in the sauce, tip in the noodles, then toss them together with the rest of the ingredients until the noodles are fully coated. Stir-fry for 1–2 minutes to heat everything through and ensure it's all mixed together.
7. Serve immediately, sprinkled with the sliced red chilli.

NOTE This is a great way to use up leftover vegetables: try adding julienned carrot, broccoli, baby corn, courgette or sugarsnap peas.

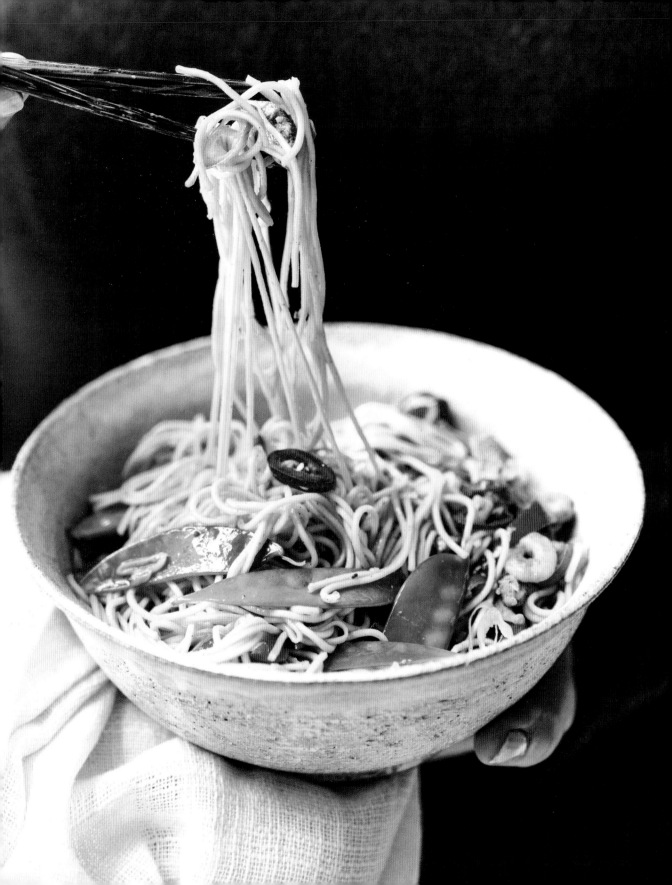

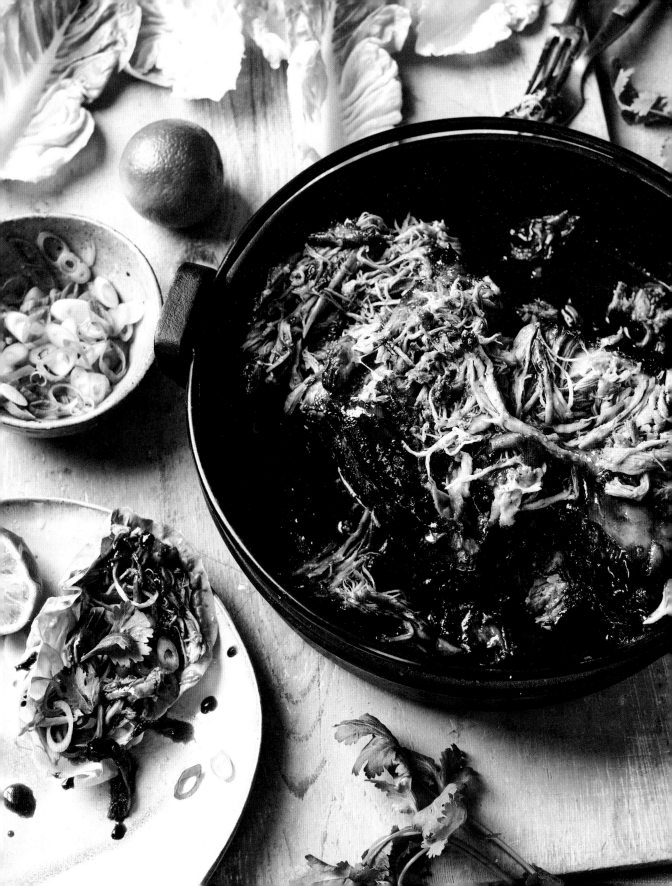

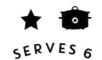

CHINESE PULLED PORK WITH LITTLE GEM WRAPS

Richly spiced, aromatic, fall-apart-tender pork is irresistibly tasty and so versatile. Serve it with rice and stir-fried vegetables, in crisp lettuce wraps or with noodles and shredded carrots.

CALORIES PER SERVING: 387

---

about 1.5kg (3lb 5oz) boneless pork shoulder, excess fat trimmed away

2 teaspoons Chinese 5 spice powder

3 tablespoons hoisin sauce

3 tablespoons dark soy sauce

2 tablespoons honey

2 tablespoons Shaoxing rice wine

1 teaspoon ground ginger

4 garlic cloves, finely chopped or crushed

2 Little Gem lettuces, bottom stalk trimmed

TO SERVE

lime wedges

sliced spring onions

handful of coriander leaves

1. Put the pork into the slow cooker bowl (it doesn't matter if some of the meat is in chunks following the removal of the fat).
2. Mix the Chinese 5 spice powder, hoisin sauce, soy sauce, honey, rice wine, ground ginger and garlic together in a small bowl, then pour over the pork and give everything a mix.
3. Pop the lid on and cook on high for 5–6 hours, or low for 10–12 hours.
4. Pull the pork apart with 2 forks, stirring it into the sauce thoroughly. Serve with lettuce leaves to use as wraps, with the lime wedges, sliced spring onions and coriander.

NOTE Shaoxing rice wine is intended specifically as a cooking wine and is a key ingredient that can be used to add fantastic flavour to many Chinese-style dishes. It is widely available, but if you are not able to get hold of it, then you can substitute with mirin, which is a Japanese sweet cooking wine.

> TO COOK THIS IN THE OVEN INSTEAD, PREHEAT THE OVEN TO 170°C/150°C FAN (340°F), GAS MARK 3½, PLACE THE PORK INTO A LARGE CASSEROLE DISH, POUR THE SAUCE OVER AND COOK IN THE OVEN (LID ON) FOR 5 HOURS. THE PORK IS READY WHEN YOU CAN PULL IT APART EASILY WITH A FORK. MIX THE SHREDDED MEAT INTO THE SAUCE BEFORE SERVING.

SLOW-COOKER MEXICAN BEEF

Beef cooked to tender perfection in a rich and aromatic Mexican-style sauce. Serve with Perfect Oven-baked Chips (see page 151) and shredded crisp lettuce, and top with cheese, jalapeños and coriander.

CALORIES PER SERVING: 293

500g (1lb 2oz) beef (such as shin or braising steak), excess fat trimmed off, chopped into chunks

1 onion, finely chopped

1 red pepper, chopped

2 tablespoons Fajita spice mix (see page 212)

1 tablespoon cornflour

400g (14oz) can chopped tomatoes

2 tablespoons tomato purée

500ml (18fl oz) beef stock

1 tablespoon red wine vinegar

400g (14oz) can black beans, drained and rinsed

TO SERVE

shredded lettuce

grated Cheddar cheese

pickled jalapeños

coriander leaves

Perfect Oven-baked Chips (see page 151)

1. Put the beef, onion, red pepper, spice mix and cornflour into the slow cooker bowl and stir it all together.
2. Add the chopped tomatoes, tomato purée, stock, vinegar and black beans. Give everything a mix.
3. Cook on high for 6–8 hours, or on low for 10–12 hours. At the end of the cooking time you can remove the lid, but keep cooking on high for 30 minutes to evaporate some of the liquid and reach the desired consistency.
4. Once cooked, break up the meat with a wooden spoon and serve scattered with shredded lettuce, grated Cheddar, jalapeños and a few coriander leaves, with homemade chips on the side.

NOTE To cook this dish in a regular oven, preheat the oven to 180°C/160°C fan (350°F), Gas Mark 4, place the ingredients in a casserole dish, cover with a lid and cook in the oven for 3 hours, removing the lid for the last 30 minutes of the cooking time.

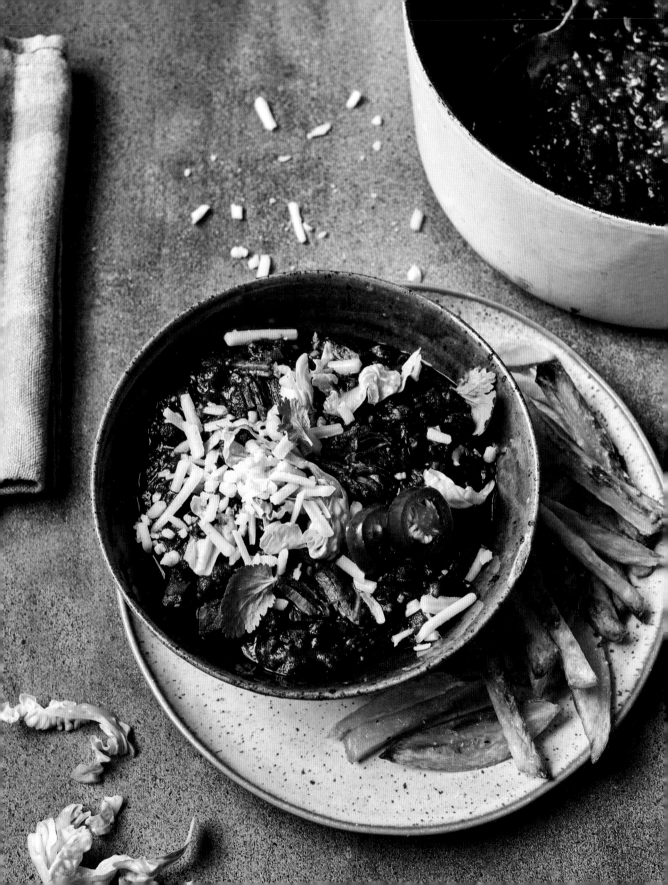

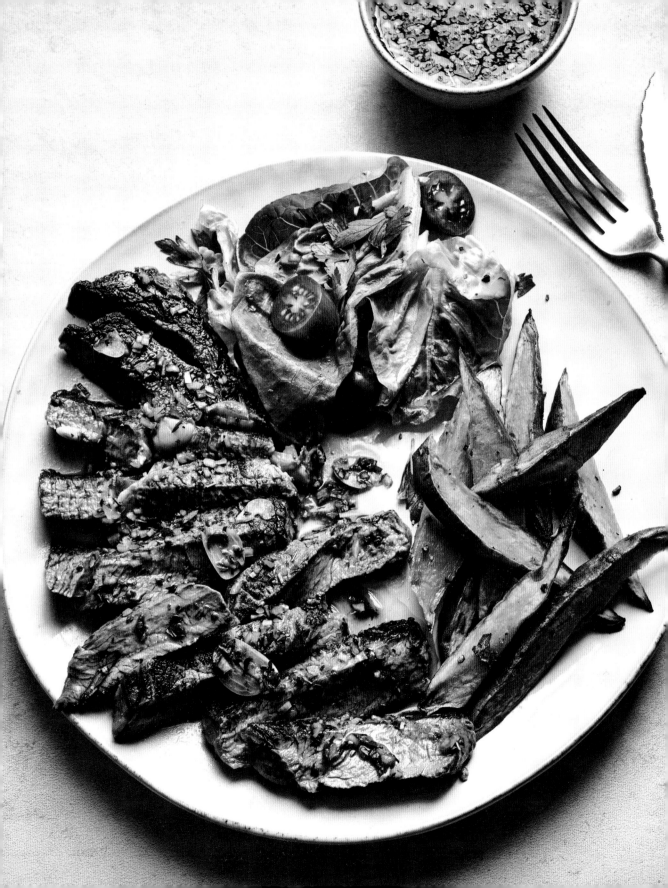

CHIMICHURRI STEAK

**Chimichurri is an Argentinian dressing that combines herbs and garlic
– it works beautifully with a perfectly cooked steak. Swap the wedges
for Perfect Oven-baked Chips (see page 151) for a classic steak dinner.**

**CALORIES PER
SERVING: 386**

2 sirloin or ribeye steaks
1 teaspoon sunflower or
    vegetable oil
coarsely ground salt and
    pepper

FOR THE CHIMICHURRI
1 shallot, peeled and very
    finely chopped
1 red chilli, deseeded and
    finely chopped
2 garlic cloves, finely chopped
5g / ⅛oz parsley leaves, very
    finely chopped, plus extra
    to serve
1 teaspoon dried oregano
½ teaspoon salt
3 tablespoons red wine
    vinegar
juice of ½ lemon

TO SERVE
mixed salad
Baked Sweet Potato Wedges
    (see page 150)

1. Take the steaks out of the refrigerator and leave at room temperature for at least 30 minutes before cooking.
2. Prepare the chimichurri by combining all the ingredients in a small bowl. Set aside.
3. Preheat the oven to a low temperature and place a large plate in to warm (for resting the steaks on after cooking).
4. Place the steaks on a separate plate and drizzle over the oil. Use your hands to rub it all over both steaks, so they are very lightly covered.
5. Place a dry frying pan over a high heat and allow it to heat up for about 1 minute before laying the steaks in the pan.
6. Keep the heat high and fry for 3 minutes, turning both steaks every minute (this is for rare steak, see note below on timing steaks).
7. Place the steaks on the warm plate from the oven, season with salt and pepper and allow to rest for about 5 minutes.
8. When you're ready to serve, plate up the steaks, spoon the chimichurri dressing over each one and serve with sweet potato wedges, a salad and extra parsley sprinkled over.

NOTE Steaks can differ in thickness and cooking times can vary, but as a general rule of thumb (for a steak around 2cm / ¾ inch thick), for a rare steak I cook it for 3 minutes, medium-rare for 4 minutes, medium for 4½ minutes and well done for about 8 minutes. Allowing the steak to reach room temperature before cooking will help it to cook evenly.

SIMPLE BAKES & DESSERTS

● ● ● ● ● ● ● ● ● ● ● ● ●

Freshly baked goods are always a temptation for me, so to strike a happy balance I love to have them as an occasional treat. This chapter contains just a few that I like, both sweet and savoury. They are healthier options, but still taste amazing. I love the scent of baking bread or cake wafting through the house and I know I cannot resist anything freshly baked, so these recipes allow me to enjoy what I've made without consuming huge amounts of calories.

The Scrumptious No-added-sugar Teabread is a regular in my household. It's a great lunchbox addition or post-school snack for my daughters and is just so easy and quick to whip up for unexpected guests. The Lemon & Blueberry Yogurt Loaf Cake was totally inspired by a slice of cake I once had from a bakery on the Isle of Skye – it was really dense and moist, not overly sweet but just so satisfying to eat. Again, this is a great one to cook when you have company.

On the savoury side, my aunt kindly allowed me to share her Auntie June's Warm Irish Wheaten Bread recipe. This has long been a family favourite due to its easy 'no knead' approach. It makes a lovely accompaniment to soup, and also the best toast with marmalade or jam. The Quick & Easy Wholemeal 3-ingredient Flatbreads are another regular in my household. I make them to go with soups, curries and stews and they are also ideal as pizza bases.

● ● ● ● ● ● ● ● ● ● ● ● ●

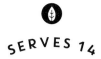

AUNTIE JUNE'S WARM IRISH WHEATEN BREAD

Dense and comforting, Auntie June's bread has been a family favourite for years. Her recipe is the easiest way to whip up delicious, home-baked bread, with no lengthy kneading and proving required. I serve it freshly baked with homemade soup, spread with Easy Chia Seed Summer Fruit Jam (see page 25) and it also makes a great base for beans on toast.

CALORIES PER SLICE: 164

225g (8oz) self-raising flour

340g (11¾oz) wholemeal flour

1 teaspoon salt

1 tablespoon caster sugar

4 teaspoons baking powder

1 teaspoon bicarbonate of soda

500ml (18fl oz) semi-skimmed milk

1. Preheat the oven to 180°C/160°C fan (350°F), Gas Mark 4.
2. Place the self-raising flour, wholemeal flour, salt, sugar, baking powder and bicarbonate of soda into a mixing bowl and stir everything together.
3. Pour the milk into the dry ingredients and mix it all together to form a wet dough (I use a table knife to do the mixing).
4. Scrape the dough into a large (900g / 2lb) loaf tin (no need to line it, as the bread slips out easily) and place on the middle shelf of the oven. Bake for 45 minutes. It will be golden brown on top and if you insert a knife it should come out clean.

NOTE This bread is at its best eaten on the day it is baked, but after that it makes great toast. If you like, you can decorate the top of the loaf before baking with porridge oats, sunflower seeds, pumpkin seeds or sesame seeds.

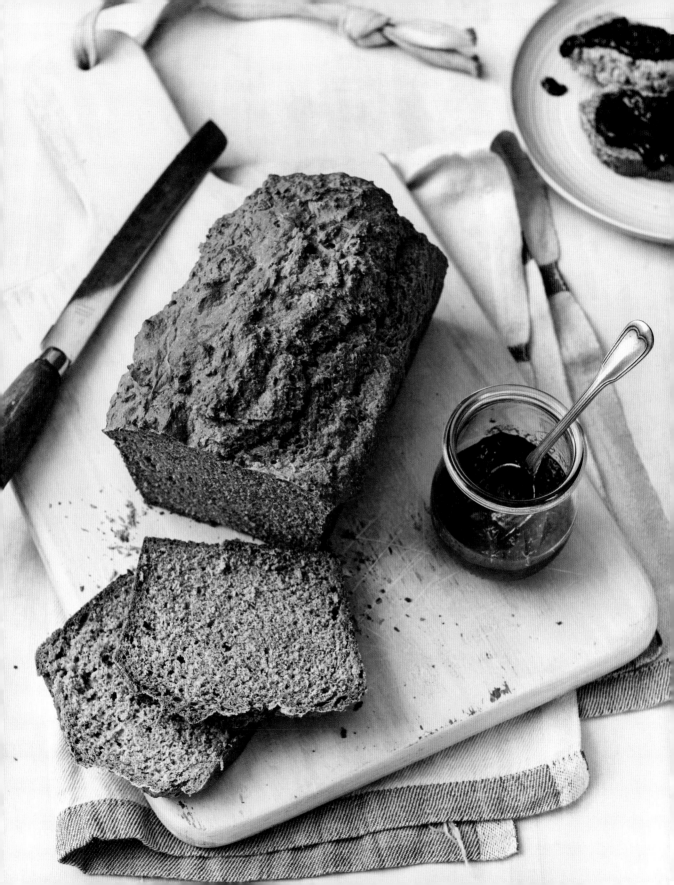

QUICK & EASY WHOLEMEAL 3-INGREDIENT FLATBREADS

These quick pan-fried flatbreads are such a useful thing to have up your sleeve. They are great with soups, salads or curries, sliced up with dips or even as a healthy pizza base. And OK, yes, 4 ingredients... but I'm not counting the salt!

CALORIES PER SERVING: 152

150g (5½oz) fat-free Greek yogurt
150g (5½oz) wholemeal flour
1 teaspoon baking powder
salt

1. Mix together all the ingredients with a pinch of salt to form a dough, give it a quick knead to make sure everything is combined, roll into a big ball, then divide into 4 pieces.
2. Roll each piece into a ball, then roll out flat to about a 15cm (6 inch) diameter.
3. Place a nonstick frying pan over a high heat, let it come up to temperature, then pop on the first flatbread. Cook it for about 20 seconds on each side: it will turn golden brown and puff up slightly. Repeat with the remaining 3 flatbreads.

NOTE You can add herbs and seasonings – such as dried oregano, nigella seeds or chilli flakes – to the flatbreads if you want to give them a little flavour. Or spread with Make-ahead Marinara Sauce (see page 214), cover with grated cheese and grill, for a quick pizza.

PASSION FRUIT, MANGO & LIME CHIA DESSERT

Bursting with tropical flavours, this is the perfect refreshing sweet dish (see photograph on page 191). The ambrosial mix of passion fruit, mango and lime in smooth, creamy yogurt is interspersed with little crunchy pops of chia seeds.

CALORIES PER SERVING: 250

100g (3½oz) mango, chopped
200g (7oz) fat-free Greek yogurt
juice of 1 lime
2 teaspoons honey
3 passion fruit
4 tablespoons chia seeds

1. Using a hand blender, or mini blender, whizz together the mango, yogurt, lime juice and honey until smooth.
2. Remove the pulp from 2 of the passion fruit and stir into the yogurt mixture. Add the chia seeds and stir to combine.
3. Spoon into 2 small glass bowls, cover and refrigerate for at least 4 hours.
4. When the desserts have set, divide the final passion fruit over the top and serve, or refrigerate until needed.

NOTE Try swapping the natural Greek yogurt for coconut-flavoured yogurt for an even more tropical taste.

LIGHTER ETON MESS

A quick, pretty and sweet dessert, perfect for a little light treat. Vanilla ice cream mixed with fat-free Greek yogurt has a lovely, whipped, creamy consistency that pairs perfectly with ripe strawberries and crunchy meringue for a dessert tasting far more indulgent than it really is.

CALORIES PER SERVING: 183

50g (1¾oz) reduced-fat vanilla ice cream

50g (1¾oz) fat-free Greek yogurt

1 meringue nest, broken into small pieces

100g (3½oz) strawberries, hulled and quartered

1. Put the ice cream and yogurt in a small bowl and mash with a fork until you have a smooth whippy 'cream'.
2. In a pretty glass or bowl, create layers of the ice cream mix, meringue and strawberries. Serve immediately.

NOTE Try this with different berries, such as blueberries and raspberries, or even some diced mango.

OPPOSITE Lighter Eton Mess (above), Passion Fruit, Mango & Lime Chia Dessert (below).

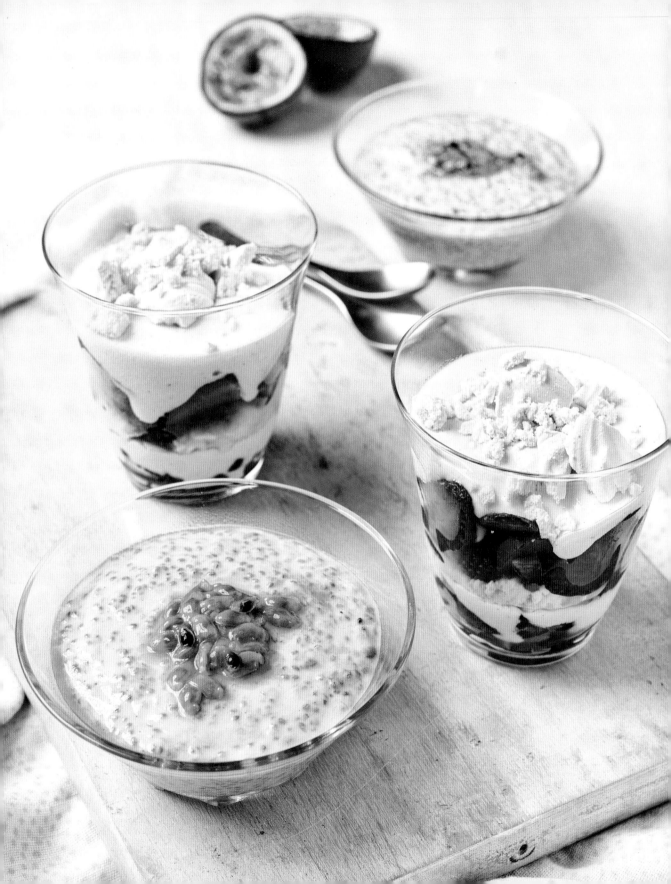

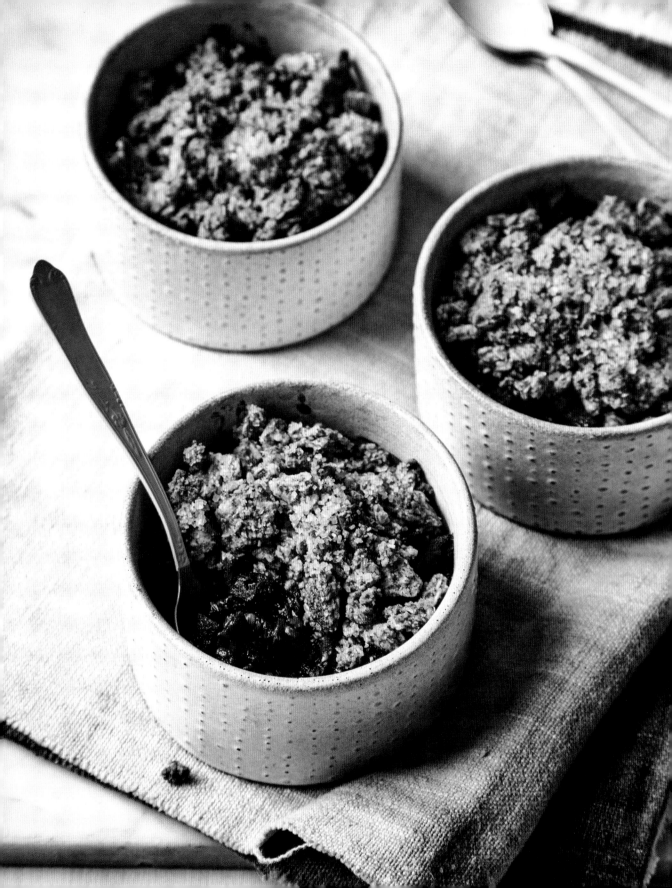

MINI BRAMBLE CRUMBLES

Warm, sweet, subtly cinnamon-spiced apples and blackberries with crunchy, golden baked oat crumble topping. The scent of warm baking crumble is one of the best in the world, and these little desserts always go down a treat.

CALORIES PER SERVING: 187

FOR THE FILLING

4 apples, peeled and
    chopped (use a sweet
    variety, such as Gala or
    Golden Delicious)
150g (5½oz) blackberries
1 teaspoon vanilla extract
½ teaspoon ground
    cinnamon
100ml (3½fl oz) water

FOR THE CRUMBLE

1 egg white
80g (2¾oz) oats
1 tablespoon maple syrup
½ teaspoon ground
    cinnamon
2 teaspoons demerara sugar
low-calorie cooking spray

1. Preheat the oven to 200°C/180°C fan (400°F), Gas Mark 6.
2. Put all the filling ingredients in a small saucepan, bring to the boil, then simmer gently for 20 minutes.
3. Meanwhile, whisk the egg white for about 1 minute until it is soft and fluffy, then stir in the oats, maple syrup and cinnamon.
4. Line a baking tray with baking parchment and spread out the oat mixture. Use the back of a spoon to flatten it out; you want it to be as thin as possible. Put the oats on the top shelf of the oven to bake for 10 minutes.
5. Remove the baking tray from the oven and allow to cool for a couple of minutes. When the oats have cooled enough to handle, break them and crumble them up with your hands as much as possible.
6. When the filling has been simmering for 20 minutes, give it a bit of a mash using a potato masher or wooden spoon, then divide between 4 ramekins. Sprinkle the crumble mixture evenly on top.
7. Sprinkle ½ tsp demerara sugar over the top of each crumble, pop them on a baking tray and bake for 10 minutes. The crumble topping will be golden and crunchy when they are ready. Serve warm.

NOTE In the UK, you find ripe blackberries in the hedgerows between July and mid-September. Many supermarkets now also sell blackberries year-round, but if you can't get hold of any, try experimenting with different mixes, such as apple and raspberry, or apple and blueberry – or just add a couple more apples for a humble crumble!

LEMON & BLUEBERRY YOGURT LOAF CAKE

Densely satisfying, moist cake with jammy bursts of blueberry and a lemony tang, this cake is incredible straight from the oven, but stays moist and delectable for 3–5 days.

CALORIES PER SLICE: 135

225g (8oz) fat-free Greek yogurt
3 eggs
100g (3½oz) caster sugar
1 teaspoon vanilla extract
finely grated zest and juice of 1 unwaxed lemon
200g (7oz) self-raising flour
250g (9oz) blueberries
low-calorie cooking spray

1. Preheat the oven to 180°C/160°C fan (350°F), Gas Mark 4.
2. In a mixing bowl, whisk together the yogurt, eggs, sugar, vanilla extract, lemon zest and juice. Fold the flour through the mixture, then stir in the blueberries.
3. Scrape the mixture into a 900g (2lb) loaf tin lined with baking parchment and bake on the middle shelf of the oven for 45 minutes. When it's ready, the cake will have risen and will be a light golden colour on top.

NOTE Try mixing up the flavours in this recipe, swapping the lemon zest and juice for orange and the blueberries for raspberries for another delicious combination.

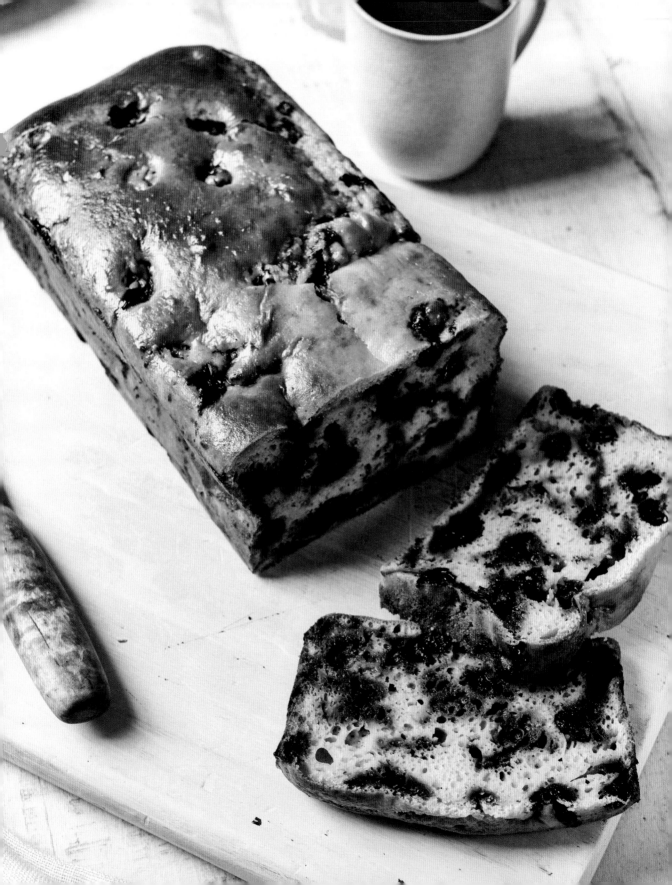

STEAMED JAM SPONGE MUG CAKE

This is a quick-hit dessert to satisfy any cake craving! Soft, warm sponge is glazed in sweet jam to give a similar consistency to a traditional English steamed jam pudding, full of nostalgic comfort.

CALORIES PER SERVING: 317

40g (1½oz) oats
1 teaspoon baking powder
1 tablespoon granulated
    sweetener
1 teaspoon vanilla extract
2 tablespoons fat-free Greek
    yogurt
1 egg
2 teaspoons raspberry jam

1. In a mini blender or a chopper, whizz up the oats to form a flour. Add the baking powder and sweetener and whizz again.
2. Add in the vanilla extract, Greek yogurt and egg and whizz until well combined.
3. Scrape half the mixture into a large mug, dollop in the jam, then add the other half of the mixture.
4. Microwave for 1 minute 45 seconds. To check it's cooked, just press gently on the top (just be careful not to burn your fingers!). It should feel firm and springy. If it's squishy, then pop it in for another 30 seconds.
5. Tip out upside-down on to a plate: the jam will be sitting on top. Eat warm.

NOTE Try replacing the raspberry jam with golden syrup or chocolate spread.

DEVONISH SCONES

The scent of baking scones is irresistible. I grew up in Devon and have a thorough appreciation of the traditional scone. Most recipes use lots of butter, but I wanted to find a version on the lighter side that was still tasty and could pass for a 'proper' Devon scone (see photograph on pages 200–1). Try these slathered with Easy Chia Seed Summer Fruit Jam (see page 25).

CALORIES PER SCONE: 65

150g (5½oz) plain flour, plus extra to dust
1 teaspoon caster sugar
1½ teaspoon baking powder
100g (3½oz) fat-free Greek yogurt
½ teaspoon vanilla extract
1 egg, lightly beaten
salt

1. Preheat the oven to 220°C/200°C fan (425°F), Gas Mark 7.
2. Combine the dry ingredients in a mixing bowl with a pinch of salt, make a well in the middle, then add the yogurt and vanilla extract. Using a metal spoon, start to mix the yogurt into the dry ingredients.
3. Once the yogurt is combined with the flour, use your hands to knead it quickly into a dough – but do not overwork the dough or the scones will rise too much when you bake them. Leave to rest for 10 minutes before rolling out.
4. Place on a lightly floured work surface and roll out to about 1cm (½ inch) thick. Using a small (5cm / 2 inch) round, fluted cutter, cut out 11 scones.
5. Line a baking tray with baking parchment and place the scones on top. Brush the top of each scone with the beaten egg and bake on the middle shelf of the oven for 10–12 minutes. The scones will have risen and will be golden brown on the outside and fluffy on the inside.
6. These are delicious served warm or cold.

NOTE To make cheese scones, omit the sugar and the vanilla extract, and add 40g (1½oz) grated mature Cheddar cheese.

CHOCOLATE ORANGE FUDGY SQUARES

Temptingly rich and dense chocolate orange slices, which use black beans instead of flour. Not only do the black beans add a fudgy texture and a dark, chocolatey colour, they are also full of fibre and protein, so are a great way to pack in those nutrients. These fudgy squares are delicious on their own, served with fresh berries such as strawberries and raspberries, or with hot custard.

CALORIES PER SLICE: 82

400g (14oz) can black beans, drained and rinsed

3 eggs

150g (5½oz) fat-free Greek yogurt

1 teaspoon vanilla extract

4 tablespoons maple syrup

2 tablespoons light brown soft sugar

finely grated zest of 2 oranges

30g (1oz) cocoa powder

½ teaspoon salt

1½ teaspoons baking powder

low-calorie cooking spray

50g (1¾oz) milk chocolate, chopped into small chunks

1. Preheat the oven to 200°C/180°C fan (400°F), Gas Mark 6.
2. In a food processor, whizz up the beans, eggs, yogurt, vanilla extract, maple syrup and sugar until smooth.
3. Add in the orange zest, cocoa powder, salt and baking powder and whizz together again until everything is thoroughly mixed.
4. Line a 20cm (8 inch) square cake tin with baking parchment and spray with low-calorie cooking spray.
5. Pour the mixture into the cake tin and scatter the chocolate chunks over the top.
6. Place on the middle shelf of the oven for 15 minutes. After the cooking time, insert a knife into the middle to check whether it's cooked through: if the mixture is still liquidy, pop back into the oven for another 5 minutes, then check again.
7. Cut into 16 squares and enjoy warm or cold. Store in an airtight container in the refrigerator for up to 5 days.

NOTE Put any leftover slices into an airtight container or sealed food bag and freeze for up to 3 months. Defrost at room temperature.

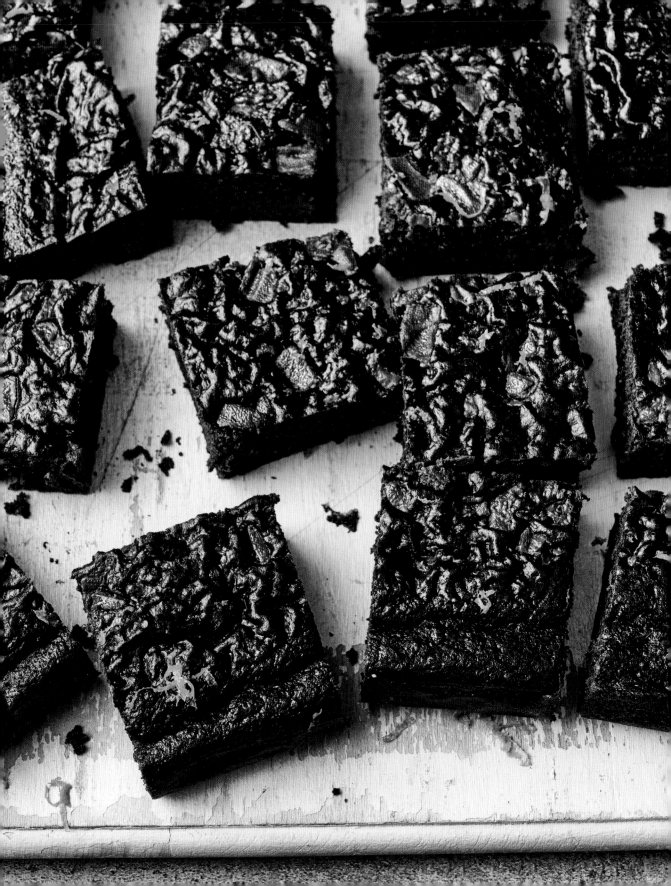

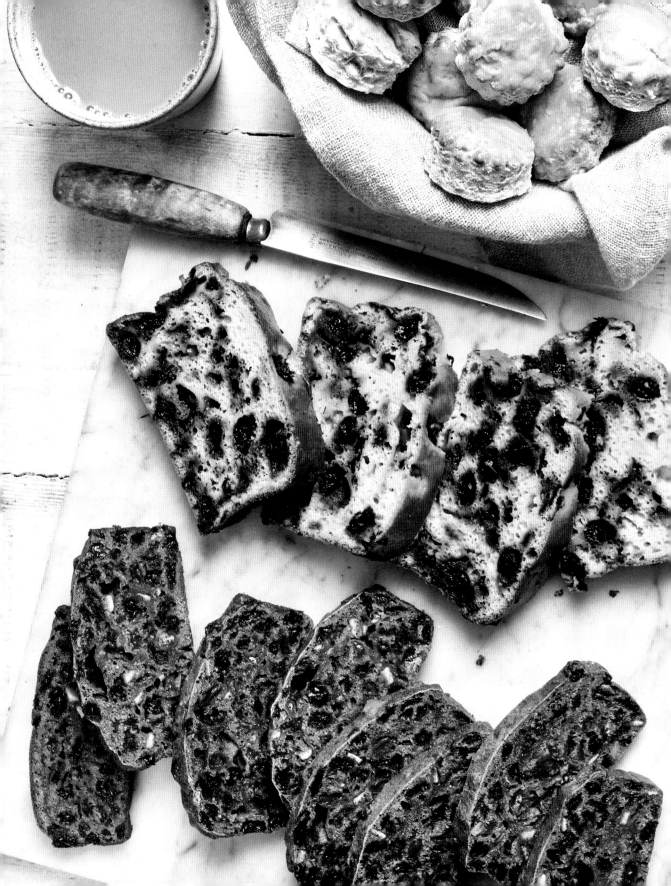

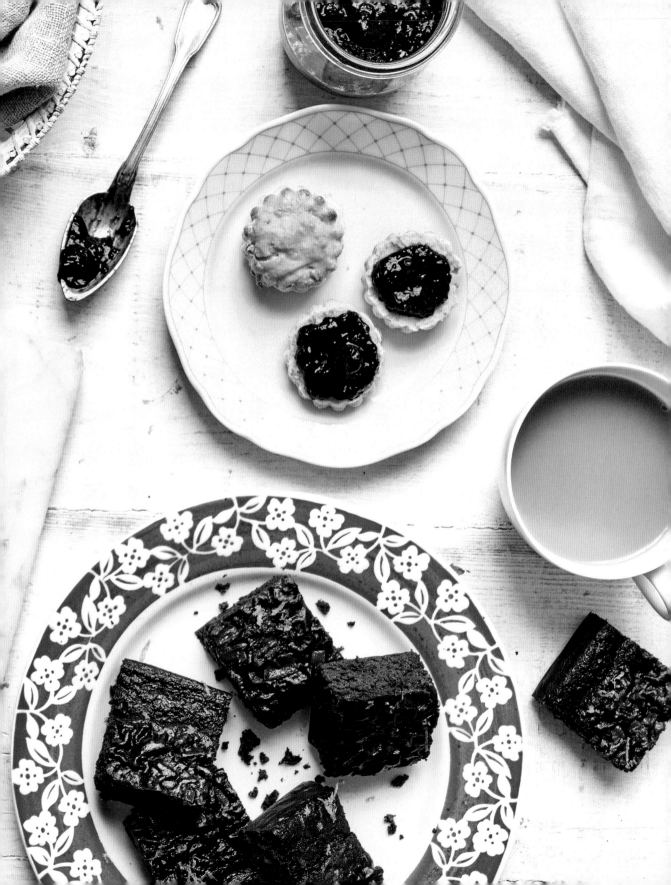

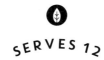

SCRUMPTIOUS NO-ADDED-SUGAR TEABREAD

I love the scent of baking teabread: warm, rich and gently spiced. The natural sweetness of the dried fruit means that there is no need to add any extra sugar. I use a half-and-half mix of white and wholemeal flour to increase the fibre content. This is lovely served warm or cold.

**CALORIES PER
SLICE: 162**

250ml (9fl oz) hot, strongly brewed breakfast tea
325g (11½oz) mixed dried fruit
1 teaspoon mixed spice
115g (4oz) white self-raising flour
115g (4oz) wholemeal plain flour
1 egg
low-calorie cooking spray

1. Preheat the oven to 180°C/160°C fan (350°F), Gas Mark 4
2. Make up the tea and allow to steep for at least 5 minutes. Put the dried fruit in a large mixing bowl, pour in the hot tea and stir. Leave for another 5 minutes.
3. Add the mixed spice, then pour in both the flours and crack the egg into the bowl.
4. Once all the ingredients have been added, mix everything together thoroughly.
5. Line a 900g (2lb) loaf tin with baking parchment, or a loaf tin liner, and spray with low-calorie cooking spray. Spoon the batter into the tin and spread out evenly.
6. Bake on the bottom shelf of the oven for 1 hour. The loaf will look browned and well-cooked on top, and will be dense but not doughy inside.

NOTE Try experimenting with different teas, such as Earl Grey or Darjeeling, for subtle flavour enhancements.

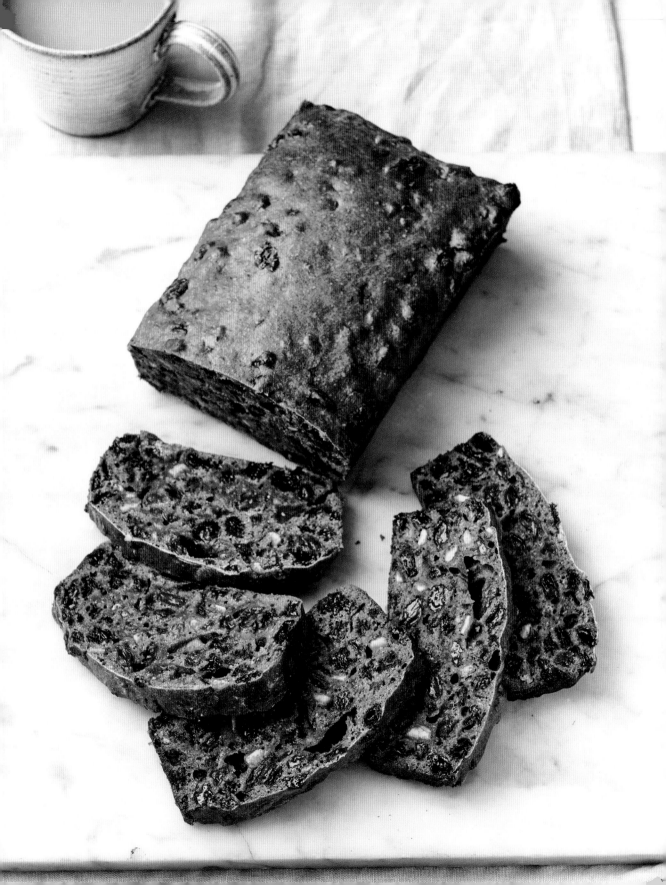

....

DIPS
DRESSINGS
SPICE MIXES
& STAPLES

....

• • • • • • • • • • • • •

I make hummus a lot! I love it as a healthy snack served with sticks of raw carrot or pepper. I also serve it with tabbouleh and falafel for a varied lunch. I'm well-known amongst my friends for always bringing a big bowl of hummus to any dinner party and I love to experiment with different flavours – my sweet potato recipe is one of the most popular! I've included a couple of my other favourite dips in this chapter too. I'm particularly proud of my Zucchimole, which I created to be a guacamole replacement, but also reminds me of the most delicious tomatillo salsa verde that I once ate in Mexico.

Having spice mixes made up in advance makes life so much easier, as I find myself using the same mixes a lot. As well as being great for the recipes suggested, they can be used as a rub to liven up any meats (also great for barbecues) and they make fantastic seasonings for sweet potato wedges, oven chips, rice or roasted vegetables as well.

The Make-ahead Marinara Sauce is something really useful to have in the fridge and I use it for all sorts during the week, such as a pasta sauce or a pizza sauce. It's so handy to fall back on when you are lacking in dinner inspiration or just need to magic something up nice and quick.

I've included two stock recipes in this chapter; stock takes time to make, but it's a great way of cutting down on food waste and adds so much more flavour to a dish than a stock cube or pot. Stock is a great thing to make when you have time, and you can simply store it in the freezer for when you need it.

• • • • • • • • • • • • •

GENTLY SPICED SWEET POTATO HUMMUS

I was so excited the first time I discovered how to make healthy hummus! I absolutely love it, as a dip with raw pepper, carrot sticks or celery, or as part of a main meal served with tabbouleh and falafel. This has a lovely creamy consistency, thanks to the sweet potato, and the slightly smoky flavour with a hint of chilli makes it temptingly moreish.

CALORIES PER SERVING: 173

2 medium-sized sweet potatoes (about 300g / 10½oz total weight)

400g (14oz) can chickpeas, drained and rinsed

1 garlic clove, peeled

200g (7oz) fat-free Greek yogurt, plus extra if needed

¼ teaspoon cayenne pepper

½ teaspoon smoked paprika, plus extra (optional) to serve

½ teaspoon ground cumin

1 teaspoon salt

juice of ½ lemon

cumin seeds, to serve (optional)

1. Prick the sweet potatoes a few times with a sharp knife and either bake them in an oven preheated to 200°C/180°C fan (400°F), Gas Mark 6, for 45 minutes, or microwave them for 7 minutes. Either way, check they are done by spearing them with a fork – it should go in easily. Slice them down the middle to allow the flesh to cool.

2. Pour the chickpeas into a food processor, then add the garlic, yogurt, cayenne pepper, smoked paprika, cumin, salt and lemon juice.

3. Scoop in the cooled sweet potato flesh (if it's still slightly warm that's fine), then blend everything together until you have a smooth and creamy consistency.

4. If the hummus is a little too thick, you can add a little bit of extra yogurt until it's the consistency you prefer.

5. If you are serving this to guests and want to make it look pretty, scoop into a serving bowl and sprinkle a few cumin seeds and some smoked paprika over the top.

NOTE A basic hummus recipe can be dressed up with so many different flavours. If you start with a 400g (14oz) can chickpeas, 1 garlic clove, 200g (7oz) fat-free yogurt, 1 teaspoon salt and the juice of ½ lemon, you can add whatever flavours you fancy – try pickled jalapeños, roasted red peppers and wild garlic – or add a spice mix from pages 212–13 to create a themed flavour to match a specific meal.

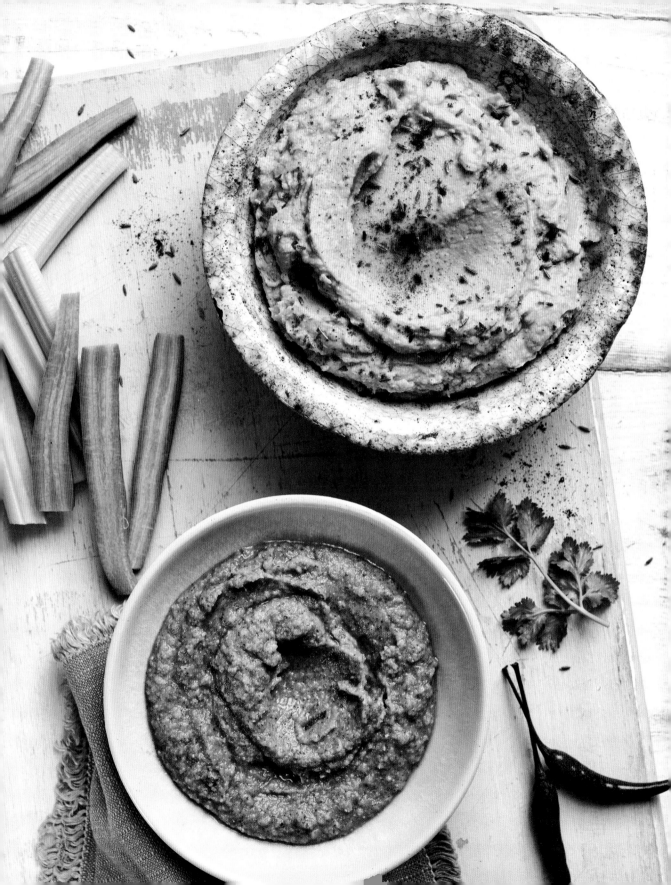

ZUCCHIMOLE

I wanted to create a copycat guacamole recipe to go alongside my favourite Mexican dishes. To get that creamy consistency, I blend cannellini beans with courgette, then use lime, chilli and coriander to get those signature flavours in. In my opinion this is just as good as guacamole. Try it with Smoky Mexican Black Bean & Sweet Potato Stew, Flaming Fajita Traybake or Weekend Veggie Chilli (see pages 58, 88 and 157).

CALORIES PER SERVING: 93

400g (14oz) can cannellini beans, drained and rinsed
250g (9oz) courgette, roughly chopped
1 garlic clove, peeled
1 green chilli, seeds removed
1 red chilli, seeds removed
finely grated zest and juice of 1 unwaxed lime
large handful of coriander leaves and stalks
½ teaspoon salt

1. Put all the ingredients into a food processor and blend until everything is combined into a smooth and delicious dip.

NOTE If you fancy a more textured dip, mash the cannellini beans with a potato masher, finely chop the courgette, garlic, chillies and coriander, and mix everything together with the lime zest, juice and salt. You could also add finely chopped tomatoes, to mix it up.

PREVIOUS PAGE Gently Spiced Sweet Potato Hummus (above), Zucchimole (below).

SMOKY BUTTER BEAN DIP

A creamy dip flavoured with smoky paprika and a hint of lemon juice. Delicious with carrot and pepper sticks, and I love to spread it lavishly on freshly cooked Quick & Easy Wholemeal 3-ingredient Flatbreads (*see* page 188).

CALORIES PER SERVING: 79

400g (14oz) can butter beans, drained and rinsed
1 garlic clove, peeled
4 tablespoons fat-free Greek yogurt
juice of ½ lemon
1 teaspoon smoked paprika
½ teaspoon dried oregano
½ teaspoon salt

1. Put all the ingredients into a food processor and whizz up until smooth.

NOTE This butter bean base is a great vehicle for lots of flavours –Try adding some roasted peppers or a fresh chilli. It's also easy to scale up this dip to feed a big group.

SERVES 2

SALAD DRESSINGS

These simple salad dressings will liven up any salad. Most salad dressing recipes contain a lot of oil, which tastes good but adds a lot of calories. But you can still get amazing flavour and a great dressing without using additional oil. It's important to dress the salad just as you are about to eat it, to keep the leaves fresh and crisp.

LIME & CHILLI

CALORIES PER SERVING: 18

A simple, hot and zingy dressing that will go with any Mexican-style salads, or to dress a simple salad alongside dishes such as Smoky Mexican Black Bean & Sweet Potato Stew, Fiesta Beef or Flaming Fajita Traybake (see pages 58, 73 and 88). This dressing is also perfect paired with my Mexican-style Bounty Bowl (see page 137).

1 teaspoon hot sauce, such as sriracha
juice of 2 limes
1 garlic clove, crushed
½ teaspoon ground cumin
½ teaspoon salt

1. Simply mix up the ingredients in a small bowl.

MISO & GINGER

CALORIES PER SERVING: 23

A salty, tangy and savoury dressing, with a delicate hint of warm ginger. Delicious over a simple salad of crisp lettuce and ribboned carrot for a Japanese-style twist. Pair this with my Japanese-style Bounty Bowl (see page 138).

1 tablespoon rice vinegar
1 teaspoon miso paste
1 teaspoon peeled and finely grated fresh root ginger
2 tablespoons light soy sauce

1. Simply mix up the ingredients in a small bowl.

WHOLEGRAIN MUSTARD

CALORIES PER SERVING: 16

A tangy, warm and subtly spicy dressing, ideal for salads and roasted vegetables. Or pair this with my English Garden Bounty Bowl (see page 139).

2 teaspoons wholegrain mustard
2 tablespoons cider vinegar
1 garlic clove, crushed
1 tablespoon finely chopped parsley leaves
salt and pepper

1. Mix together the mustard, vinegar, garlic and parsley in a small bowl, then season to taste with salt and pepper.

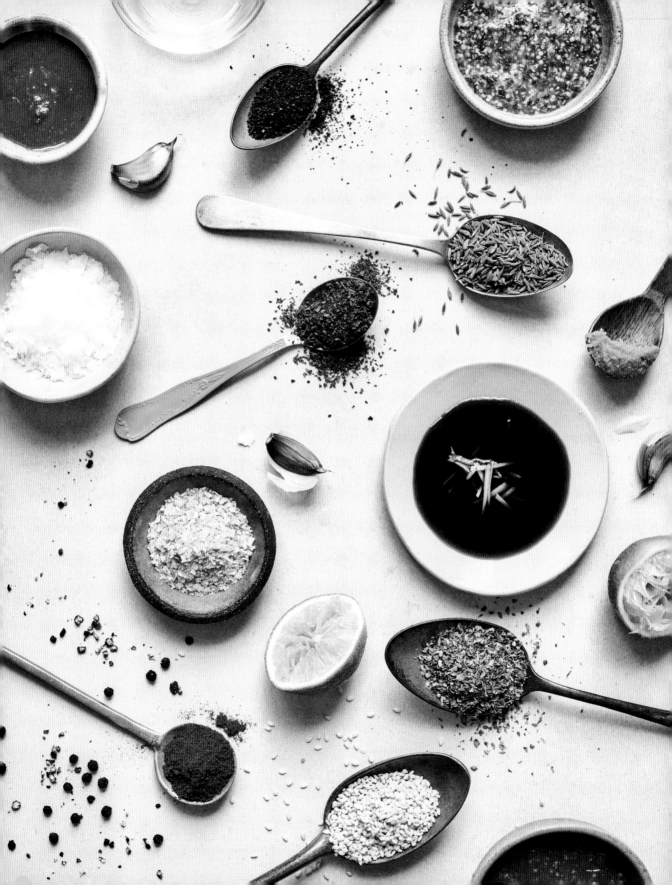

SPICE MIXES

I always have some spice mixes made up at home, as I find it makes life so much easier than measuring out individual spices every time I make a certain meal. I use these mixes often – in traybakes, as a quick coating for fried chicken, as a rub to liven up any meats (great for barbecues) and to make fantastic seasonings for sweet potato wedges, oven chips, or even just rice or roasted vegetables. I make up the mixes in cleaned-out empty jam jars. They are quick and easy to pull together and a great time saver.

TACO

MAKES ABOUT 10 TABLESPOONS

2 tablespoons garlic granules
2 tablespoons onion granules
2 tablespoons paprika
1 tablespoon chilli powder
1 tablespoon dried oregano
1 tablespoon ground cumin
1 tablespoon salt
1/2 tablespoon pepper

1. Combine all the ingredients and store in a jam jar or other airtight container.

NOTE Use this in Fiesta Beef (see page 73).

FAJITA

MAKES 13 TABLESPOONS

2 tablespoons chilli powder
2 tablespoons smoked paprika
2 tablespoons ground cumin
2 tablespoons dried oregano
2 tablespoons garlic granules
2 tablespoons onion granules
1 tablespoon salt

1. Combine all the ingredients and store in a jam jar or other airtight container.

NOTE Use this in Flaming Fajita Traybake and Slow-cooker Mexican Beef (see pages 88 and 180).

PERI-PERI

MAKES 9 TABLESPOONS

1 tablespoon paprika
1 tablespoon onion granules
1 tablespoon garlic granules
1 tablespoon granulated sweetener
1 tablespoon ground coriander
1 tablespoon chilli flakes
1 1/2 teaspoons salt
1 1/2 teaspoons pepper
1 1/2 teaspoons dried parsley
1 1/2 teaspoons dried oregano
1 1/2 teaspoons cayenne pepper
1 1/2 teaspoons ground cumin

1. Combine all the ingredients and store in a jam jar or other airtight container.

NOTE Use this in Peri-peri Chicken with Sweetcorn Salsa (see page 165).

ZA'ATAR

**MAKES ABOUT
15 TABLESPOONS**

3 tablespoons sesame seeds
4 tablespoons dried oregano
4 tablespoons dried marjoram
3 tablespoons sumac
1 tablespoon cumin seeds
½ tablespoon salt

1. Fry the sesame seeds in a dry frying pan for a couple of minutes until they are lightly toasted and just starting to pop.
2. Pour into a jam jar or other airtight container, add the rest of the ingredients and shake to mix.

NOTE Use this in Za'atar & Orange Roast Chicken with Lemon Roast Potatoes (see page 110).

CAJUN SEASONING

MAKES 13 TABLESPOONS

2 tablespoons smoked paprika
2 tablespoons dried oregano
2 tablespoons Italian seasoning
2 tablespoons garlic granules
1 tablespoon onion granules
1 tablespoon cayenne pepper
1 tablespoon dried thyme
1 tablespoon pepper
1 tablespoon salt

1. Combine all the ingredients and store in a jam jar or other airtight container.

NOTE Use this in Cajun Chicken Rainbow Rice (see page 55).

MAKE-AHEAD MARINARA SAUCE

Make this up ahead of a busy week and keep it in the refrigerator and you have a brilliant start for lots of easy meals. This rich, tomatoey pasta sauce will beat anything you can buy. It's also perfect on pizza or can be stirred into cooked mince and onions to make a delicious quick Bolognese. Simply make a batch, pour into a large jar and keep in the refrigerator ready for when you need it.

CALORIES PER SERVING: 85

4 garlic cloves, crushed
2 × 400g (14oz) cans chopped tomatoes
1 tablespoon tomato purée
1 carrot, roughly chopped
2 teaspoons dried basil
1 teaspoon dried oregano
1 teaspoon salt
¼ teaspoon pepper
200ml (7fl oz) water

1. Simply put all the ingredients into a deep saucepan, bring to the boil, give everything a good stir, then leave to simmer for 40 minutes.
2. After the cooking time, blitz the sauce, using a hand blender or a food processor, until smooth, then transfer to a large (1 litre / 1¾ pint) jar. Allow to cool, then keep in the refrigerator for up to 5 days. If you don't use it all up, put what's left into portion-sized pots in the freezer for when you need it.

NOTE For a hands-off approach, you can make this in a slow cooker. Just put all the ingredients into the bowl and cook on high for 4 hours, or low for 8 hours. You can also leave the sauce chunky if you prefer, rather than blending it at the end.

BALTI 'SAUCE FOR EVERYTHING' CURRY

I love having a go-to sauce to use up leftover roast meats, or vegetables that need eating up. This simple sauce is great with leftover chicken, lamb, beef or turkey. It can also be turned into a delicious vegetarian curry by adding peppers, cauliflower, potato, chickpeas or anything else you fancy. Just make up the sauce and add in a bit of whatever you have in the refrigerator or storecupboard.

CALORIES PER SERVING: 88

1 teaspoon garam masala

1 teaspoon ground cumin

1 teaspoon ground coriander

1 teaspoon mustard seeds

½ teaspoon ground cinnamon

low-calorie cooking spray

2 onions, finely chopped

2 garlic cloves, crushed

5cm (2 inch) piece of fresh root ginger, finely chopped

2 red chillies, deseeded and finely chopped

400g (14oz) can chopped tomatoes

250g (9oz) tomato passata

juice of 1 lemon

1 teaspoon salt

1. Mix the ground spices together in a small bowl.
2. Spray some low-calorie cooking spray into a sauté pan or deep frying pan and add the onions. Fry over a medium heat for 8 minutes, stirring occasionally.
3. Add the garlic, ginger and red chillies to the pan and stir-fry for 1 minute. Add the spices and stir-fry for a further 30 seconds.
4. Tip in the chopped tomatoes, then fill the can with water and add that too. Pour in the passata and add the lemon juice and salt, stir everything together and simmer for 30 minutes.
5. Now you can make any additions that you like. If you are adding leftover meat, ensure you heat it through thoroughly. If you are adding a quick-to-cook vegetable, such as cauliflower, or canned chickpeas, you can just add these to the pan, put a lid on and simmer for about 10 minutes. If you are adding potato, you will need to pre-cook it before adding.

NOTE If you don't have leftovers to use up, you can just make this into a chicken balti. Once you have made the sauce, simply add 3–4 chicken breasts and poach them in the curry sauce for 30 minutes while it is simmering. You can then remove the cooked chicken and slice it up, or just break it up with a wooden spoon into the curry.

VEGETABLE STOCK

Homemade stock can add so much extra flavour to food and it's a great way to use up odds and ends of vegetables that you might otherwise discard. The ingredients below are only a loose guide, as you can add in what you have and still have a delicious stock (for example, if you don't have all the herbs, just use what you do have). Avoid starchy vegetables such as potatoes, parsnips and turnips, or bitter vegetables such as broccoli, cauliflower and green beans.

CALORIES PER 100ML (3½FL OZ): 9

1 onion, quartered
2 celery sticks, sliced
1 leek, trimmed, rinsed and sliced
4 chestnut mushrooms, quartered
2 carrots, tops removed, roughly chopped
a few parsley sprigs
2 thyme sprigs
2 bay leaves
8 peppercorns
1.4 litres (2½ pints) cold water
1 teaspoon salt

1. Put all the ingredients except the salt into a large saucepan and bring to the boil. Reduce the heat to a simmer and cook gently, uncovered, for 1 hour.
2. Add the salt, stir it through, then strain the stock through a colander into a large bowl or plastic container. If you'd like it completely clear, then also strain it through a sieve to remove any small particles.
3. Keep in the refrigerator or freezer for when it's needed.

NOTE I pick out the peppercorns and bay leaves, then put all the cooked vegetables from the stock into a freezer bag or container. I freeze these and use them to add lovely extra flavour to future soups. A great way of saving on waste too.

CHICKEN STOCK

I always try to get the most out of a roast chicken by making a stock with the carcass. This creates a great base for so many recipes and means that nothing goes to waste. It's also a great way to use up slightly past-it vegetables! This can be used in Thai Chicken Noodle Soup, Cajun Chicken Rainbow Rice (see pages 52 and 55) or as the base for a chicken gravy.

CALORIES PER 100ML (3½FL OZ): 17

1 leftover chicken carcass
1 onion, skin on, quartered
3 carrots, tops removed
2 celery sticks
2 litres (3½ pints) water
1 teaspoon salt
¼ teaspoon pepper
1 rosemary or thyme sprig
  (or whatever herbs you
  have in)

1. Put all the ingredients except the salt into a large saucepan and bring to the boil. Reduce the heat to a simmer and cook gently, uncovered, for 3 hours.
2. Alternatively, you can cook this in the oven. Preheat the oven to 180°C/160°C fan (350°F), Gas Mark 4, and cook with a lid on for 3 hours.
3. Strain the stock through a colander into a large bowl, then strain through a sieve into another bowl or container.
4. Keep in the refrigerator for up to 4 days, or freeze (you can do this in silicone muffin moulds for easy portions).

NOTE Make a tasty soup from the vegetables that you cooked in the chicken stock, rather than throwing them away. Simply use a hand blender to whizz the vegetables up with some of the stock, and then add any leftover chicken meat and any desired veg (try peas, carrots or potatoes) and simmer together until the vegetables are cooked. Delicious!

> **IF YOU WISH TO REMOVE THE FAT FROM THE COOKED STOCK, ALLOW IT TO COOL COMPLETELY SO THE FAT RISES TO THE TOP AND SETS – THIS CAN THEN BE EASILY REMOVED AND DISCARDED.**

FREEZER-FRIENDLY MEALS

NOTE ON PASTA

When you freeze a pasta dish, the defrosted and reheated pasta will be a little more 'mushy' than when you first made it. Denser, smaller pasta shapes, such as macaroni, freeze better than spaghetti.

QUICK & EASY MIDWEEK MEALS

ONE-POT WONDERS

SAVOURY TRAYBAKES

FAMILY FAVOURITES

LIGHT DISHES & SIDES

FRIDAY NIGHT SPECIALS

SIMPLE BAKES & DESSERTS

DIPS, DRESSINGS, SPICE MIXES & STAPLES

GLOSSARY

UK	US
aubergine	eggplant
back bacon rashers	lean bacon slices, such as Canadian-style bacon
baking parchment	parchment paper
baking tray	baking pan or baking sheet
beef, shin or braising	beef, shank or chuck
beetroot	beet
bicarbonate of soda	baking soda
borlotti beans	cranberry beans
broad beans	fava beans
brown sauce	steak sauce
butter beans	lima beans
caster sugar	superfine sugar
chestnut mushroom	cremini mushroom
chilli flakes	dried red pepper flakes
chips	French fries
cider	hard cider
chopping board	cutting board
coriander	cilantro (unless ground and referring to the seed)
cornflour	cornstarch
courgette	zucchini
crumble	crisp (the dessert); crumb (the topping)
egg, large	US super-large egg
fish sauce	Thai fish sauce
grill, grill pan	broiler, broiler pan (noun); broil (verb)
haricot beans	navy beans
hob	stove
jacket potatoes	baked potatoes
jug	liquid measuring cup or pitcher
jumbo oats	old-fashioned oats
flaked almonds	slivered almonds
kitchen paper	paper towels
lamb neck fillet	boneless lamb shoulder
loaf tin	loaf pan; a 900g/2lb pan is about 23 x 13 x 7cm (9 x 5 x 3 inches)

UK	US
mangetout	snow peas
minced beef	ground beef
mixed spice	allspice
pak choi	bok choy
passata	tomato puree or sauce
pepper (red pepper)	bell pepper
pizza base	pizza crust
plain flour	all-purpose flour
pork fillet	pork tenderloin
porridge	oatmeal
porridge oats	rolled oats
prawns (king)	shrimp (jumbo)
pulses	legumes
rocket	arugula
salad leaves	salad greens
self-raising flour	use all-purpose flour plus 1 teaspoon baking powder per 125g (4½oz) of flour
semi-skimmed milk	low-fat milk
sieve	strainer
spring onion	scallion; green onion
steak, sirloin	steak, tenderloin
stock	broth
stock cube	bouillon cube
storecupboard	pantry
summer fruit mix	raspberries, strawberries, blueberries and/or other berries of choice
sweetcorn	corn kernels
takeaway	takeout
tenderstem broccoli	broccolini
tomato purée	tomato paste
traybake, savoury	baked in a casserole or roasting pan
whizz	to process in a food processor or blender
wholemeal flour	whole-wheat flour

INDEX

ABOUT THE AUTHOR

Pip lives in Devon with her husband and two young daughters, juggling food-blogging and family life. After studying English Literature at Cardiff University, Pip lived in London for 10 years, working in Human Resources. Pip has always had a passion for food and cooking for friends and family. After returning to Devon in 2012, she set up The Slimming Foodie blog in 2015 to share healthier takes on her favourite dishes.

www.theslimmingfoodie.com
@the_slimming_foodie

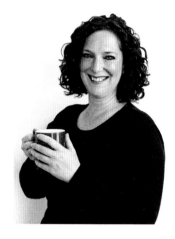

Author photograph by Darren Vincent

AUTHOR'S ACKNOWLEDGEMENTS

I never expected that I would be writing my first cookbook during a global pandemic, and it certainly brought some extra challenges! A huge thank-you to my husband and best friend, Darren, who has been by my side for the best and the worst times, kept me calm during moments of panic in the intense recipe-testing and writing process, and added so much creative input into The Slimming Foodie. Thank you to my two incredible kind, caring and clever daughters, Miette and Marlie, for being so patient and understanding during the months when my attention was focused on the book, for bringing me cups of tea and lavishing me with endless hugs. I am so proud of you both. Thank you to my parents, Val and Brian, for always being there for us.

Thank you to the whole team at Octopus, who have brought this book together during the most challenging of times: Natalie Bradley, for her huge enthusiasm and faith in The Slimming Foodie, and for listening to our vision throughout the process; Sybella Stephens and Yasia Williams for all of their hard work. Thank you also to everyone that I haven't been able to meet but who have also put so much into the book: Peter Dawson, Amy Shortis, Lucy Bannell, Sarah Reece, Lucy Carter, Nic Jones, Karen Baker, Hazel O'Brien and Kevin Hawkins.

To my agent, Heather Holden-Brown, for believing in me from our first conversation and for holding my hand through the unfamiliar process.

Also, a huge thank you to the shoot dream-team – your talent and efficiency had me in awe and you all made the shoot such great fun. Chris Terry for the incredible photography and a relaxed and upbeat approach (and keeping us well fed!), Tamsin Weston for the fantastic props styling, Henrietta Clancy for the beautiful food styling and huge task of cooking all of the dishes, and Olivia Somary for being a brilliant assistant.

Last, but definitely not least, thank you to everyone who follows The Slimming Foodie blog and social media channels – every like, comment, share, save and view makes a difference, and I'm so appreciative of this lovely community.